Eating Disorders

EVERYTHING YOU NEED TO KNOW

REVISED EDITION

JIM KIRKPATRICK, MD

AND PAUL CALDWELL, MD, CCFP(C)

FIREFLY BOOKS

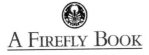

A FIREFLY BOOK

Published by Firefly Books (U.S.) Inc. 2004

Copyright © 2004 by Jim Kirkpatrick and Paul Caldwell

All rights reserved. No part of this publication may be reproduced, stored in a retrieval system or transmitted in any form or by any means, electronic, mechanical, photocopying, recording or otherwise, without the prior written permission of the publisher.

First Printing

Publisher Cataloging-in-Publication Data (U.S.)

Kirkpatrick, Jim.
    Eating disorders : everything you need to know / Jim Kirkpatrick, Paul Caldwell.
Rev. ed.
[208] p. : ill. ; cm.
Includes index.
Summary: Expert advice on the causes, effects and treatment of anorexia nervosa, bulimia nervosa, binge-eating and other eating disorders.
ISBN 1-55297-976-8 (pbk.)
1. Eating disorders -- Diagnosis. 2. Eating disorders – Treatment. 3. Anorexia nervosa -- Treatment. 4. Bulimia -- Treatment. I. Caldwell, Paul. II. Title.
616.85'26 dc22   RC552.E18.K55 2004

Published in the United States in 2004 by
Firefly Books (U.S.) Inc.
P.O. Box 1338, Ellicott Station
Buffalo, New York 14205

Published in Canada in 2004 by Key Porter Books Limited.

Design: Peter Maher
Electronic formatting: Heidy Lawrance Associates

Printed and bound in Canada

To my loving wife, Gail,
who submitted this manuscript
in its embryonic state,
and my kiddies, Paul and Amy,
whom I love to bits.

J.K.

To my daughters,
Jen, Amy, Lucy and Nina—
you lift me up
with your love.

J.P.C.

———————

Shelley, Erin, Christine,
Jennifer, Alison and Leane—
our loving memory of you
is what keeps us dedicated.

The quotation from Thomas Morton is from "A Treatise on Consumption," published in 1694. The quotation from Sir William Gull is from "Anorexia Nervosa (Apepsia Hysterica, Anorexia Hysterica)," a paper presented to the Clinical Society of London in 1873. The quotation from Charles Lasègue is from "De l'anoréxie hystérique," published in 1873.

Contents

Preface

In another life I was a musician. I performed with many popular and jazz groups and toured with a show group for several years. We had singers, dancers and a band with brass instruments, string instruments, keyboards, drums and guitars. I played bass guitar and flute. We toured 275 days of the year, did some recording and had our own national television series.

One day it became evident to me that one of the dancers was not well. She had lost a lot of weight, to the point of being emaciated. In spite of this, she remained charming and vivacious and able to meet the demands of rigorous dance rehearsals and performances. Later in life I asked someone who had known her what kind of illness she had been dealing with, and was told, "She had anorexia nervosa."

Around the same time I was performing with this group, the media were peppering the news with stories of Karen Carpenter and her struggle with anorexia nervosa. These stories took me back to a time when I visited A&M Recording Studios in Los Angeles. Richard and Karen Carpenter were in the studio; they were the most successful recording artists for A&M Records at the time, and I could barely afford a cup of coffee. When rumors of Karen's eating disorder emerged, I couldn't help but ask myself how someone so successful could develop such a devastating disorder, which would eventually take her life. It made me wonder, "Where could this kind of condition come from, and why?"

It was in medical school that I first became part of the care of someone with an eating disorder. I worked on the psychiatric wards and met several young women admitted because of their struggles with anorexia nervosa. I was moved by the grip this disorder had on them, but I had a sense of helplessness, not knowing what I could do for them.

During an outpatient psychiatric rotation, I saw a young woman diagnosed with bulimia. This delightful young woman very kindly told me how she could eat such excessive quantities of food and then purge. The session left me amazed and bewildered.

While working on one of my medical elective classes, where I adapted high-tech musical instruments for the physically disabled, I visited the Juilliard School in New York City. Waiting to meet the dean of the school, I noticed the thinnest girls I had ever seen. They were young ballet students. I wondered how they could even stand, let alone dance.

Without my realizing it, these experiences were sensitizing me to the plight of those with eating disorders, and their families. In fact, these events were setting the stage for me to become a caregiver and political advocate for those with eating disorders.

After graduating from medical school and becoming established in family practice, I met a young patient who seemed to have *both* anorexia nervosa and bulimia. She was extremely thin but would vomit frequently. She had almost every medical complication an eating disorder could cause. She impressed upon me the destructive nature of eating disorders, and made me acutely aware of the need for effective, humanitarian treatment options.

Since then, I have been part of the care of several hundred people with one form of eating disorder or another. For my first few years in private practice I worked as an eating-disorders intensivist, following some patients very closely on a day-to-day basis. I was required to do a lot of crisis intervention, from a medical perspective as well as to prevent suicide and other self-harm. I was involved with these patients' therapy, medical management, nutrition and family support, in the community as well as in the hospitals. I worked with children, adolescents and adults. It was through my involvement with all these people and their families that I developed my understanding of eating disorders. Today I am involved with a wonderful community-based multidisciplinary eating-disorders treatment team that works to meet the challenges that eating disorders bring.

Not only was I involved as a clinician, but I became interested in advocacy. Because of a great need for more treatment facilities locally and throughout the province, I helped establish the British Columbia Eating Disorders Association. Soon after, I joined the Provincial Steering Committee on Eating Disorders and became chair of the board. I was especially interested in seeing what could be done about improving the education of caregivers in the area of eating disorders. Being on the editorial board of the professional journal *Eating Disorders: The Journal of Treatment and Prevention* gives me a first-hand look at what researchers are doing around the world to provide better treatment and prevention options. I am also a member of the Academy for Eating Disorders (AED), an international society of professionals dedicated to improving the care of those with eating disorders. Through the AED I am attempting to stimulate further interest in the education of professionals in the various healthcare disciplines. This book is a stepping stone toward that goal.

The single most important thing I have learned over the years is that individuals with eating disorders do recover. For that reason, this book is ultimately one of optimism and hope for those who have these disorders, and for their families and friends.

Jim Kirkpatrick, M.D.

In medicine, some diseases are much easier to understand than others.

Strep throat, for example, is quite straightforward. We know that it is caused by the bacterium *Streptococcus*, that we get it from someone else by droplet spread, and that it is fairly simply treated with antibiotics. The whole concept of the disease and its treatment is universally recognizable, something we can all easily grasp.

But other diseases, such as eating disorders, are not like this at all. They are complicated, mysterious processes that, though very common in our society, have elements that are foreign to most of us. Diseases in which people starve themselves to skeletal thinness, or vomit huge quantities of food they have eaten in binges, have aspects that are not within the realm of experience for most of us. We cannot easily identify with the feelings and actions. In addition, there are so many unknowns, so many theories and speculations, that it's hard to grasp the concepts and the particulars of treatment. How can we understand these events? How can we sympathize with these feelings? How can we help?

This book is written, in all its detail, to answer these questions. It's written to give you knowledge about these problems, and information to begin the process of recovery. We believe in recovery. We believe it's possible, and we believe you believe in it too.

The book begins with an introduction, a beginning perspective on these complicated illnesses, then proceeds to describe anorexia, bulimia, binge-eating disorder and others in detail, emphasizing the complex mix of physical and emotional factors involved. Eating disorders often do not exist alone, and other factors (such as depression, drug and alcohol use, etc.) are explained in Chapter 4, "Factors That Complicate Eating Disorders." Chapter 5, "Understanding Eating

Disorders," focuses on the cultural, genetic and personal forces that initiate and then perpetuate these problems. Chapter 6, "Medical Treatment," and Chapter 7, "Medications That May Help," bring to light different medical options including the use of medications. Chapter 8, "Psychological Treatment," reviews what psychological approaches have been found to be helpful, and what to expect from therapy. The final chapter, "The Road to Recovery," shows what the recovery process looks like, emphasizing that recovery is a real, obtainable goal.

Whether you yourself have an eating problem, or someone you love has one, we sincerely hope that this book helps— helps you cope, helps you understand these sometimes bewildering processes, and helps give you strength—strength you will need on the journey toward recovery.

Paul Caldwell, M.D.

Acknowledgments

Over the years, I have learned everything I know about eating disorders through contact with other people. In particular I owe deepest gratitude to the people whose care I have been part of—people who have lived the challenges of an eating disorder, and their families.

I would like to thank the professional team with which I work at the Eating Disorders Program in British Columbia's Capital Region: Maria Tilroe, Peggy Folkes, Susan Boegman, Sharon Watson, Catherine Carr, Carol Tickner, Sherry Gale, Claire Winterton, Gabriele Ratjen, Marianne Le Claire, Janice Briggs, Dawn Olson, Dr. Lori Vogt, Dr. Cliff Duncalf and Dr. Richard Stern. Our office support staff—Debra Sigurdson, Vikki McDonald, Valerie Trace, Laura Workman and Kathryn Cowan—are appreciated more than they know. I very much appreciate working with Diane Kay, Joanna Parkin, Andrea Lemp, Regan Tuppert, Dr. Chris Deroche and all the staff of Duncan Mental Health. Many thanks to the hospital staff I have worked with over the years, often in very difficult situations. In particular I would like to thank the staff of the Eric Martin Pavilion and pediatric wards of Victoria General Hospital who have stayed the course. I also value the support of the Ministry for Children and Families and the Ministry of Health of British Columbia. The province and I owe much to the British Columbia Eating Disorders Association for its role in advocacy and education. The support given to the province by the St. Paul's Eating Disorders Program and the British

Columbia Children's Hospital Eating Disorders Program is greatly appreciated.

I have been fortunate enough to work with many individuals who have been dedicated, over the years, to improving the care of people with eating disorders: Dr. Laird Birmingham, Linda Lauritzen, Dr. Elliot Goldner, Dr. Pierre Leichner, Vicki Smye, Dr. Roger Tonkin, Dr. Winston Mahabir, Dr. Ron Manley, Ardis Brown, Dr. Terry Russell, Dr. Keith Sigmundson, George Whitman, Elizabeth Cull, Sonjia Franklin, Stephanie Ustina and Heather McKenzie. I am also fortunate to be working with Françoise Juneau and staff of the Lester B. Pearson World College of the Pacific.

The Provincial Eating Disorders Program thanks Sarah McLachlan for giving her support to our cause.

Thanks to Lynne Parten, Laura Reinhardt, Astrid St. Pierre, and Sarah McKenzie for their input.

A debt of gratitude is owed to the Academy for Eating Disorders, now under the direction of Dr. James Mitchell, for uniting the world of professionals who care desperately for those they serve.

Thanks to Dr. Paul Caldwell, and to Anna Porter of Key Porter Books, for endless endurance through the development of this book. Thank you to my wife, Gail Kirkpatrick, for submitting the manuscript in the first place.

I would like to thank my partners and staff at Colwood Corners' Physicians for being such a dedicated team.

I very much appreciate being permitted to work on this manuscript for many hours at Olive Olio's Pasta and Espresso Bar and Bean Around the World.

Last but not least I must thank my dear friends of the Freak Brothers Corporation, who keep me grounded, and in particular Professors Alan Mitchell, Don Wilkes and Bob Mitchell, who introduced the world to the concept of addiction management.

J.K.

Introduction

The relationship we have with food is not at all a simple one, but rather a complicated, multi-faceted connection to this biological necessity.

From an infant's suckling of breast milk, through the difficult years of teaching toddlers to eat properly, and on into adult life, our choice of food and our relationship to our choices are central to our daily existence.

All of us have experienced hunger—that uncomfortable feeling somewhere in the abdomen that is eliminated by eating. We live in a time of such excess that, if we experience hunger at all, it's a brief disturbing symptom, an inconvenience only, often occurring simply because of poor planning. Our ancestors knew a different kind of hunger—a much more powerful and threatening anguish that persisted for days or weeks on end and would not be quieted. Hunger was a threat to their lives, a powerful physical signal of inadequate nutrition, and it screamed at them, day after day, from the hollows of their bodies.

Why We Eat What We Eat

Most people in the developed world realize, at least on an intellectual level, that we need an adequate volume and variety of food to survive. We understand the necessity of eating food from various groups to ensure balanced nutrition, but we choose our foods not only because of their nutritive value, but also because of the sensual pleasure they offer. The smell of fresh-perked coffee, the crunch of an apple, the frozen sweetness of ice cream, the tingle of a fresh orange slice are all examples of the huge variety of pleasures food can provide.

Eating is also a social phenomenon. It is the focus of our daily mealtime gatherings. It's an acceptable break from work and a time to share with family or friends.

Food is often associated with festivity and reward. The feasts of earlier times have now evolved into the turkey dinner "with all the trimmings" we eat at holiday time, the birthday cakes we serve our children and the thousands of "special" meals we serve each other as celebrations or symbols of love. On an individual basis, food is often used as a reward or for solace, as a comfort in times of stress or distress. Somehow the feeling of fullness, of satiety, of giving in to the food we eat, is associated with feelings of peace, calm and relief from anxiety. Our eating and our emotions are closely connected.

For every society and in every culture, certain foods have been forbidden, for either social or religious reasons, and others have been encouraged. Christians ate fish on Fridays, not because of any inherent nutritional value of fish as a food, but to remind them of Jesus, who said to his disciples, "I will make you fishers of men." The Judaic and Muslim tradition of avoiding pork and eating only food that is kosher or halal may have originated in an attempt to avoid illnesses carried in pork, but now is enforced as a confirmation of faith. Around the world, certain foods are associated with good luck, prosperity and success. Clearly, we find many values in food apart from its nutrition.

When Things Go Wrong

For some people, particularly some young women, this relationship with food changes and becomes quite abnormal. Their attitudes to food, their food choices and their eating become disordered, producing a group of medical problems (such as anorexia nervosa and bulimia) referred to as eating disorders. Food is no longer seen as a daily requirement whose acquisition is pleasurable. Rather, it becomes something to be feared or dreaded and hence avoided (as in anorexia nervosa), or a forbidden temptation that, though not enjoyed, cannot be denied (as in the case of bulimia). The emotional turmoil inside is reflected in abnormal eating. These are not simply problems of eating, but rather problems of feeling.

One of the most difficult challenges in approaching eating disorders is understanding what is actually happening in the minds of these sufferers. Our understanding must begin with an appreciation of the complexities of our normal relationship with food. From this starting point we can begin to unravel the interwoven psychological and physical abnormalities that define these eating disorders.

People from any cultural or ethnic background can have an eating disorder. Though these disorders do occur in males, most (90 percent) occur in women, especially young and adolescent women. The disorders produce a progressive change in personality that eventually affects both the physical and the mental well-being of the sufferer.

There are four main eating disorders. Anorexia nervosa is a disorder of self-starvation in which marked weight loss is seen, as a result of either severe restriction of diet, or some mechanism (such as vomiting) to prevent food from being properly absorbed. Bulimia nervosa is a disorder in which bouts of extreme overeating are followed by deliberate vomiting or purging by some other means (such as laxatives or diuretics), or by periods of fasting. Binge-eating disorder consists of repeated episodes of overeating (bingeing) not frequently accompanied by vomiting, purging or fasting. The so-called not otherwise specified group of eating disorders includes all behaviors of eating and attitudes toward food that are considered abnormal but do not fit into the strictly defined medical diagnoses mentioned above.

Eating disorders happen to good people, young people, full of promise and potential, and they happen without the young people either choosing them or being able to control the process. An anorexic is no more able to prevent her eating disorder than someone with pneumonia is able to recover completely from the disease without medical intervention.

Eating disorders happen in good families, in which the parents truly care for their children, love them with all their hearts and have done their best to nurture them.

Why do these disorders happen? There is no easy answer to this question. These are complex and often confusing afflictions, and the processes that initiate and then perpetuate them are complicated, with powerful yet concealed forces that effect change in an invisible manner.

Usually, a combination of factors contributes to someone's abnormal relationship with food, and then the new relationship alters the individual, reinforcing itself and pushing the

What do people feel their disorders are about?

"They're about control, fear, problems of identity (especially issues that arise from being a woman and the demands and expectations projected at a woman), and our culture's obsession with image and a narrowly defined 'beauty.'"

"They're about not honoring the self. They're about fear and isolation."

"Insecurity."

"An obsession to be thin. I was overweight in my childhood and my teens. I hated it. I went on diets and lost and regained weight several times before my eating disorder began. I liked the attention I got when I was thin, especially when I got too thin—although I didn't think I was thin enough. No matter how trim I got, I liked my body. At last I had control over something. At least, I thought I did."

person away from those around her. Somehow, changing their basic relationship to food is appealing to these young people—it allows them to go somewhere, to achieve something, that was not possible before. Changing the relationship, adjusting it, makes some difference in their lives, a difference that is somehow better, and thus the behavior persists, contributing to a further sequence of events that defines the illness.

It is possible for most of those with eating disorders to be helped. However, it's very difficult to know exactly how to help—what to do, what to say, how to behave, how to show love, how to direct them towards recovery—in short, how to begin to help disentangle the bewildering knot of feelings and perceived failures. Helping these people does not come intuitively. It's not enough to reach inside yourself and feel the power of your own love, and extend that out to them, even though it's impossible not to try.

To help, to really help, demands an understanding of the circumstances and influences that initiated the disorder, and the factors and forces that perpetuate it. Without such an understanding, recovery does not take place, and lives are wasted. If you yourself have an eating disorder, or if someone you love suffers from one, reading this book will be, at the very least, a beginning step on the road to recovery.

ONE

Anorexia Nervosa

Cheryl was only 13 years old when she began her first diet.

She had always been a happy and athletically gifted child and, although she excelled in several sports, her favorite was gymnastics. She particularly enjoyed tumbling routines, the combination of lithe acrobatics with dance. One day after a practice, her coach commented that the girls on the team had bodies that were changing. He told them that they had to be careful not to become, as he put it, "too fat for gymnastics." The comment wasn't directed to Cheryl specifically, but when she left the gymnasium that day she was determined to lose some weight.

She was pleased when her dieting quickly resulted in the loss of several pounds and, though the coach didn't notice the difference, Cheryl announced to the other gymnasts a few weeks later that she had been on a diet and that she had been quite successful—she'd lost eight pounds (almost four kg) over the last month! Many of the other girls were jealous of her success, though openly they praised her. Cheryl felt good about herself, pleased that she could so easily control her appetite to achieve the desired weight loss so quickly, simply by choosing her foods more carefully.

Cheryl didn't really have a specific target weight in mind—she just continued the diet over the next few weeks—but soon her relationship with food changed. Before her diet, she had been a typical teenager, a good eater but not too discriminating. She had been equally content enjoying her mother's Sunday roast beef dinner or grabbing a hamburger and fries at the mall with her friends. But now it seemed that the specifics of food became much more important to her. By careful studying, she was able to learn about the relative nutritional values of various foods, and to identify which foods were high in fat and carbohydrates. She divided food into "good" and "bad" categories. "Good foods" were those that had very little in the way of fat or calories. She allowed herself these. "Bad foods" were high in fats and calories, sugars and salt. She avoided these. She became much more involved in food preparation than she ever had been before, insisting on doing the shopping herself, carefully picking out the family's vegetables and other produce. She began to cook the family meals, not just simple ones, but complicated affairs. Even though she would spend much of the day preparing a meal for the family, she herself didn't eat a lot of what she had made—because, of course, she was on a diet.

Food and the particulars of her diet became a major part of her life. She enjoyed this, and she saw the obvious results of her efforts in continuing weight loss. She was very careful with her food, and gradually developed a daily routine. For breakfast she restricted herself to two cups of herbal tea without sugar. Lunch consisted of a plate of carrot sticks, celery and other fresh vegetables, followed by fresh fruit such as an apple or orange. Supper consisted of steamed fresh vegetables and herbal tea, with crispbreads and low-fat yogurt. She drank only pure spring water, even in her herbal tea. She didn't snack between meals and, because of the particulars of her diet, she almost never ate away from home, except when she took her "meal" with her.

She continued to lose weight and this still pleased her, as she was obviously able to master this problem of being "too fat." On a daily basis those around her, especially her girl-friends, would remark how envious they were of her and her weight loss. She felt very special because of these comments. She weighed herself frequently on the bathroom scales, often four or five times a day. In spite of the fact that she was five feet (1.5 m) tall and weighed only 96 pounds (44 kg), she still felt that she had quite a lot of weight to lose. She checked herself in the mirror almost every night before bed, turning around to examine her thighs and buttocks in the reflection, pinching her skin to see how much fat there was. Although she had lost a lot of fat, she felt there was quite a bit yet that had to go.

She began exercising more vigorously, trying to lose more weight. She started jogging as a means of "keeping fit," and became quite dedicated to it. She would run a three-mile (five km) route around her neighborhood every morning, before her herbal tea breakfast and the first weigh-in of the day.

After a while she seemed to lose interest in the gymnastics team and, in spite of phone calls from her coach, she missed the regular team practices and competitions. When her father asked her about it, Cheryl replied that she was keeping up her fitness with her running.

She had been quite a popular student at school, with a wide circle of friends, both male and female, but now she spent most of her time alone in her room, doing schoolwork, or outside jogging to try to keep her weight down. Her parents became concerned. Although they didn't like to confront Cheryl directly, they admitted to themselves that she was a different person than she had been before puberty. They hoped it was just a stage she was going through, because they found her not nearly as likable a child, not as approachable or as easygoing as she had been. They felt that she was not as happy, and that they were unable to help her. She had become more distant, more withdrawn, from them and from the rest of the family. Her parents had, of course, expected changes to occur at this age, but they were alarmed by the nature of the changes. It was as if they were gradually and slowly losing their daughter and were powerless to influence her.

One day when Cheryl had just finished a shower, her mother entered her daughter's bedroom and saw the young girl only partially covered by a bath towel. She was shocked to see how gaunt and thin her daughter looked without the baggy clothes she usually wore. Cheryl's legs were pencil-thin, and her ribs were showing as thick, bony lines in her tiny chest. She looked frail and helpless, like a starving child. Cheryl's mother was very frightened.

"Cheryl, look at you!" she said. "You look terrible! You're so dreadfully thin—are you sick?"

"No, Mom," said Cheryl, "I'm fine. I just feel better if I'm thin."

Despite her objections, Cheryl's parents insisted that she see their family doctor, who diagnosed the girl's problem as anorexia nervosa.

The Diagnosis

Anorexia nervosa is a chronic debilitating illness in which a person demonstrates an altered eating pattern and subsequent weight loss. It is not an easy illness to understand; it is a complicated mixture of emotional, psychological and physical changes. Some aspects of the illness, such as the marked weight loss, are obvious at first glance, but these physical changes have been produced by psychological and emotional factors that are far less evident. The abnormal psychology that initiates the physical changes can best be understood as an attempt by the anorexic to control his or her life. By rigidly denying such a basic human need as food, the anorexic feels able to direct his or her own future, to be completely in charge of his or her own life. This control, demonstrated by continuing weight loss, is very important to the anorexic, and it becomes a positive reinforcement to continued, severe dieting. Unfortunately, marked weight loss by itself produces feelings of accomplishment in anorexics, and these changes reinforce the original desire for control. The psychological and emotional changes initiate the physical ones, but then the physical changes reinforce the negative psychological changes. This feedback mechanism perpetuates the disease and makes it very difficult to separate the physical changes from the psychological ones, to understand either the illness or its treatment. In spite of this complexity, however, researchers have identified a number of aspects of the disease, all of which must be part of the clinical picture before a diagnosis of anorexia nervosa can be made.

How Does Anorexia Nervosa Begin?

The onset of the illness may follow some stressful life event. This event will unlikely be catastrophic, such as the loss of a parent or the breakup of the family unit, but will more often be due to a less visible stressor—such as entering puberty, leaving home to attend school, being embarrassed or ashamed, doing poorly in school or not being allowed to participate in a chosen social group. Low self-esteem is often at the heart of these stresses. Some form of dieting to lose weight always occurs at the beginning of anorexia nervosa, and this is thought to be the mechanism through which the disease becomes evident. Almost all girls diet at some time during their adolescence, and many find the experience unrewarding and difficult. Most young women find dieting too much of a struggle. They cheat or give up before reaching their goal, abandoning their diets quickly, happy to have lost a few pounds—if indeed they have been lucky enough to do so. Because they find dieting such a futile and frustrating experience, they generally stop their food restriction after a short period of time.

However, some young women are much more successful at dieting. Their loss of weight is soon visible to their own eyes, and to the eyes of others. Because thinness is so worshipped in our society, these young girls quickly receive positive reinforcement from their friends and from the rest of society, which intensifies their desire to lose weight. They feel good about themselves and this new endeavor. They focus on the particulars of their diet, deciding on specific foods to avoid (such as fries or fatty foods); they identify some foods as allowed and some as forbidden. They are gratified by their success and energized by the positive feedback they receive daily. Here is something they can do really well! Emotionally, they feel better—they become the envy of their friends, and feel they have achieved mastery over their own bodies and their fates. They feel a sense of triumph, a gratification in this control; they are good at losing weight and, naturally, they continue to diet, enjoying their special ability to master their hunger and thus control their lives. They relish the envious comments of their friends, and the praise and approval of society. Eventually, however, their dieting and the resulting weight loss begin to inflict a series of physical changes on their bodies and minds. These changes, coupled with the increasing sense of control over their lives that successful dieting has given them, perpetuate the pattern and lead to progressive emaciation.

What's Wrong in Anorexia Nervosa?

Marked Weight Loss

In all cases of anorexia nervosa, the most striking physical sign is that the total weight of the person is significantly below what would be considered normal for his or her height and age. Normal weights, for all ages and heights, are standard measurements that have been developed through analysis of data from millions of people. In anorexia nervosa the person's weight is at least 15 percent lower than would be expected. Not only is the weight low, but the weight is maintained at this abnormally low level, or continues to fall.

Because the illness often affects young people who are still growing, actual weight loss may not occur. If a young person fails to put on appropriate weight during growth spurts (for example, fails to make an expected weight gain during a period of growth such as puberty) and, as a result, is less than 85 percent of the normal weight for his or her age and height, this too falls within the diagnostic criteria for anorexia nervosa.

Abnormal Attitude to Weight and Abnormal Perception of the Body

People with anorexia nervosa have an abnormal mental outlook with regard to their own weight, and thus to their food (which they see as the instrument of weight control). We all know that in our society it is not desirable to be obese. However, anorexics have a powerful desire to be abnormally thin. They don't want to weigh at the normal level but, rather, to weigh markedly less than the norm. This attitude, this psychological force, is very important in understanding how the illness progresses: it is the power that initiates the diet. When dieting is successful, this mindset activates the person's will to

BMI Chart

Estimating Your Body Mass Index (BMI)			

Weight

lb   kg

Women   BMI   Men

340 — 150
320 — 140
300 — 140   70
280 — 130
260 — 120   60
240 — 110

220 — 100   50   55
      — 95
200 — 90
190 — 85   40
180 — 80
170 — 75   Obese   Obese   60
160 — 70
150 —   30   Overweight
140 — 65   Overweight
130 — 60   Acceptable
120 — 55   Acceptable   20   65
110 — 50
100 — 45   70
95
90 — 40
85   75
80 — 35   10
75
70   195
65 — 30   80
60   205
55 — 25   210
50   85

Height

in   cm

50 — 125
   — 130
   — 135
55 — 140
   — 145
   — 150
   — 155
   — 160
   — 165
   — 170
   — 175
70 — 180
   — 185
   — 190
75 — 195
   — 200
80 — 205
   — 210
85

Mark your weight with a dot on the vertical line on the left. Mark your height with a dot on the vertical line on the right. Using a ruler, connect the two dots. The point where your line crosses the center (BMI) line indicates what range your weight falls into.

continue dieting to an excessive and destructive degree. Thus people with anorexia must starve themselves to satisfy their powerful mental need to be thin. Most people who diet stop when their goal is reached. Anorexics will not stop dieting.

Not only do anorexics have an overwhelming desire to be very thin; their perception of their own bodies is also markedly altered. When they examine themselves, they often feel that they still weigh too much, even when they are quite under-weight; they "see" themselves differently than others do. In spite of being alarmingly wasted and gaunt, they insist that their bodies have "too much fat." The combination of this abnormal desire to be thin and the failure to recognize that they are *not* fat maintains their overwhelming desire to deny their appetite and decrease their food intake. They identify fat as the enemy, and they see it everywhere. It isn't just that anorexics' attitude toward fat is different—they feel more strongly than most people that fat is harmful—but that somehow their whole viewpoint has changed, so that identi-fying fat and removing it (or controlling it) has become the single most important thing in their lives. The combination of this abnormal psychological drive and the altered percep-tion of their own bodies is the reason why anorexics cannot, on their own, stop the pattern of progressive weight loss. They do not have control over their weight loss. Their pathologi-cal drive for thinness has control of them.

Other Physical Changes

One of the commonest other physical changes that occurs in women as a consequence of anorexic starvation and weight loss is the cessation of menstrual bleeding. This physical sign is called amenorrhea. Because 90 percent of anorexics are women, amenorrhea has become an important physical sign by which doctors identify serious cases of the disease. A small amount of weight loss will not usually cause amenorrhea, but

Medical criteria for the diagnosis of anorexia nervosa

- a weight that is at least 15 percent lower than normal for height and age
- an unreasonable, overwhelming fear of becoming overweight or fat which persists in spite of the person being significantly underweight
- the perception that the body is overweight or fat when it is significantly underweight, or refusal to admit that the weight loss is a serious problem
- in menstruating females, the absence of at least three consecutive menstrual periods

Anorexia nervosa is further classified into two subgroups, depending on which method the person uses to restrict eating. The first type is called the "restricting type." In this subgroup, the marked weight loss has been achieved by simply restricting the food consumed by strict dieting, without any other mechanism (such as misuse of laxatives, self-induced vomiting, etc.).

The second type of anorexia nervosa is that of the "binge-eating/purging type." In this group of anorexics, the marked weight loss has been achieved by the person regularly engaging in some sort of purging behavior (such as self-induced vomiting, the misuse of laxatives, diuretics or enemas), to compensate for binge eating.

a marked weight loss almost always does so. In this case the loss of menstruation may be a reflection of how severely the body's functions have been affected by starvation. Amenorrhea can also develop as a result of psychological factors alone, because the hormones necessary to produce regular menstrual flow are affected by mental stress. In this case amenorrhea may *precede* significant weight loss. In many cases, amenorrhea is a result of a combination of psychological stress and weight loss. Of course, other causes of loss of regular menstrual flow (such as pregnancy) must be ruled out.

Anorexic or Not?

Doctors and psychologists have devised a set of criteria that a person must fulfill to be diagnosed as having anorexia nervosa. This medical definition of the disease is very important, as it allows professional caregivers to identify anorexia nervosa accurately, and to compare treatments in groups of patients, all of whom have similar signs and symptoms of the disease. Researchers understand that many people have some but not all of the symptoms of anorexia nervosa, as defined by these strict criteria; although some of these cases are severe, the medical diagnosis of anorexia nervosa does not apply to them. For example, if a young woman has an inappropriate attitude to her own weight and has not menstruated for several months, but is only 10 percent below her ideal weight, she is not medically diagnosed as having anorexia nervosa. She has not fulfilled the strict criterion of being 15 percent below the norm for her height and age. Those patients who fulfill only some of the criteria for the disease are understood to be at risk for developing the full-blown syndrome. However, they are diagnosed as having an eating disorder "not otherwise specified." This classification system may

Is anorexia nervosa inherited?

There is no doubt that anorexia nervosa runs in families. In his historic description of the disease in 1870, a physician in London, Sir William Gull, noted that "often there is something queer in the family history." More recent studies have shown that there is an increased risk of anorexia nervosa in first-degree relatives (parents, siblings or children) of individuals with the disorder. Such relatives have a ten-times-higher incidence of the disease than the general population. In addition, there is an increased incidence of mood or emotional disorders (such as depression or manic-depressive illness) in first-degree relatives of people with anorexia nervosa.

Studies of twins also suggest a genetic predisposition or tendency to the disease. Identical twins have exactly the same genetic material in their bodies. If one identical twin develops anorexia nervosa, the chance of the other twin developing the disorder is about 55 percent. However, if the twins are not identical but fraternal—that is, with differing genetic material—and one of the twins develops anorexia nervosa, the chance that the second twin will develop the illness is only 7 percent, approximately the incidence expected for any other first-degree relative.

seem clumsy and arbitrary, but it allows caregivers to make accurate comparisons between groups of patients with the more serious disease.

"Anorexia Nervosa" As a Medical Term

The word "anorexia" comes from the Greek *an*, not, and *orexis*, desire. It is used to describe the loss of desire for eating. The word "nervosa" comes from the French word *nerveux*, meaning "having to do with the nerves"—that is, having a psychological cause.

Literally translated, the term "anorexia nervosa" means "loss of appetite caused by psychological illness." The term is a misnomer. Usually, especially early in the course of the

---

The science of hunger

Although we all experience hunger sometime during our lives, it is not an easy feeling to describe in words. Some people describe hunger in terms of a desire, need, craving or appetite for food. Others call it a discomfort, pain or weakness caused by the need for food. Some of the physical sensations associated with hunger are dizziness, weakness, shaking and various gut symptoms such as gurgling or gnawing.

Hunger is a natural body sensation that signals the need for nutrition. It is created by a complicated set of mechanisms involving our thoughts, senses, stomach, intestines, hormones and brain.

Just the thought of food can trigger hunger. How often have you become hungry by looking at food advertisements in magazines or on television? Thoughts of eating can also emerge from cultural expectations to eat at certain times of the day and in certain social settings.

Some of the strongest signals for hunger come from our senses. The visual appeal of food, and its smell, can trigger hunger. Taste and texture further signal the gut and brain to be ready for food. Your ability to smell significantly affects how much you can taste, and affects your level of desire for food. As you age, your ability to taste and smell decreases somewhat, and may help to diminish your desire for certain foods. Family and cultural patterns of eating also play a major part in what makes food appealing or not appealing to us.

A strong signal for hunger is a drop in the blood glucose (blood sugar) level. When we eat, nutrients are converted into a form of sugar in the blood, so that the blood can transport this source of energy to various body parts. The hypothalamus, a part of the brain, senses the glucose level in the blood. When the level drops too low, the brain recognizes the need for more food, and senses hunger. In addition, hunger increases as the brain levels of the neurotransmitters noradrenaline, neuropeptide and corticosterone increase in response to a drop in blood glucose. (Neurotransmitters are substances that affect the transmission of messages from one nerve cell to another.)

How do we lose our feeling of hunger? When the levels of blood glucose and amino acids (broken down from the protein in food) are elevated, the brain can recognize the need to stop eating. When the stomach is stretched by food entering it, and the process of emptying the stomach slows down, the stomach sends a signal to the brain further indicating that the body has enough nutrition. Oils or fats in the stomach can help to signal that it's time to stop eating. Hormones such as cholecystokinin, which comes from the pancreas, tell the brain that the body now has adequate food. The brain responds to its own neurotransmitters, serotonin and dopamine, in monitoring food intake, and tryptophan, the amino acid from which serotonin is synthesized, can also decrease appetite.

Normal fullness (*satiation*) is the physical feeling of having enough food in the stomach. But the body senses that it has had adequate nutrition not only by this fullness sensation but also by all these other signals. *Satiety* is the overall inhibition of hunger and further eating that arises as a consequence of food ingestion. In some individuals with an eating disorder, the threshold for fullness is inappropriately low; they feel full after very small, inadequate amounts of food. Others must ingest large amounts of food to feel full.

disease, patients with the illness have not lost their appetites at all—in fact, their appetites are extremely strong and present at all times. Rather, anorexics learn to control their appetites, not give into them, and thereby control their lives. Thus the weight loss is not initially due to loss of appetite but, rather, due to strict denial of that most basic of body instincts: hunger. As the disease progresses, however, many anorexics eventually *do* lose their appetites.

Early Descriptions of Anorexia Nervosa

Although many details of the disease have only recently begun to be understood, anorexia nervosa is not a newly discovered medical problem. The essentials of the illness were documented at least three centuries ago. At that time, physicians were used to seeing the severe weight loss of many chronic diseases such as tuberculosis or cancer. The term "consumption" was used to describe the very obvious muscle wasting seen in these patients (patients were literally "consumed" by the disease until they wasted away and died). In 1689, an English physician named Thomas Morton wrote a textbook on consumptive diseases, including in it a case of "Wasting Disease of Nervous Origins" that is probably the earliest description of anorexia nervosa. He describes an 18-year-old woman who

> in the month of July fell into a total suppression of her monthly courses [menstruation] from a multitude of cares and passions of her mind, but without any symptom of ... sickness following upon it.... I do not remember that I did ever in all my practice see one, that was conversant with the living so much wasted with the greatest degree of a consumption, like a skeleton clad only in skin, yet there was no fever ... only her appetite was diminished ... and she was after three months taken with a fainting-fit and died.

Morton considered the condition "nervous consumption" and believed that it was caused exclusively by "sadness and cares." He used the term "consumption" to describe the marked weight loss, and he called it "nervous" because he could not find a physical cause (such as tuberculosis) to explain the wasting.

In the 1870s Sir William Gull and Dr. Charles Lasègue, a Parisian neurologist, published papers on a number of cases of self-starvation that are now clearly recognizable as anorexia nervosa. Gull coined the term "anorexia nervosa" to distinguish the disorder from tuberculosis, just as Morton had tried to do two centuries before. Gull felt that the disorder resulted from "a morbid mental state" and a "perversion of the ego" and that it caused the young girls whom he described to deliberately decide not to eat, and to stubbornly persist in this pursuit in the face of increasing ill health and dramatic emaciation. Gull's first patient "complained of no pain, but was restless and very active. This was in fact a striking expression of the nervous state, for it seemed hardly possible that a body so wasted with disease could undergo the exercise which seemed agreeable. There was some peevishness of temper and a feeling of jealousy. Occasionally for a day or two the appetite was voracious, but this was very rare and exceptional," and most of the time she had "complete anorexia for animal food, and almost complete anorexia for everything else." His colleague Lasègue, whose cases were almost identical, decided that the anorexia must be "hysteria," a common psychiatric grouping of female neurotic disorders at the time. Lasègue was impressed with the mental state of the patients: "what dominates in the mental condition of the hysterical patient, above all, is the state of quietude, I might almost say a condition of contentment, truly pathological. Not only does she not sigh for recovery, but she is not ill-pleased with her condition not withstanding all of the unpleasantness it is attended with."

Cases were reported toward the end of the nineteenth century and into the twentieth century. At one point the disease was felt to be due to damage to the pituitary gland (called Simmonds' disease, after the physician who first described the premature aging, loss of hair and regression of the genital organs seen in young women after damage to the pituitary). In the early part of the twentieth century, anorexic patients were treated with various hormonal injections including thyroid extracts and insulin. Later, when it became clear that Simmonds' disease was a separate condition, psychiatric explanations were offered as a cause for anorexia nervosa. We now understand that the illness is a complicated combination of physical and psychological factors, with the psychological factors initiating the problem, and both the physical and psychological factors perpetuating it.

Medical Consequences of Anorexia Nervosa

Weight Loss
Most anorexics achieve a weight 15 percent below the accepted norm for their height and age by severely decreasing the amount of carbohydrates and fat in the diet. They allow themselves only a small amount of protein daily, and many foods (such as carrot sticks and celery) that have fiber but not much nutritional value. They often maintain their vitamin intake with vitamin supplements. This type of self-willed starvation, employing a diet that is lacking in carbohydrates but includes some protein, produces a pattern of weight loss that is different from that seen in situations where adequate nutritious food is simply not available, such as famine. In the latter situations it is usually protein-rich foods that are lacking; carbohydrates may still be present in adequate amounts. When protein is lacking in the diet, marked muscle wasting occurs but it is usually combined with a swollen, distended stomach area and an accumulation of excess fluid in the legs, a condition called *kwashiorkor*. During the 1985 Ethiopian famine, we were shocked by television images of gaunt, spindly-legged infants, their huge, swollen bellies a vivid contrast to their pencil-thin limbs. The weight loss seen in anorexia produces the same muscle wasting and

the same accumulation of fluid in the legs, but there is no distension of the abdomen.

The medical term used to describe profound weight loss is *cachexia*. The word comes from the Greek (*kakos*, bad, and *hexis*, a habit of body). Cachexia is seen in many medical conditions, such as cancer and chronic infections, and it involves the loss of mainly muscle mass and subcutaneous fat. This is the type of weight loss seen in anorexia nervosa; it produces a skeletal appearance that is quite striking.

The normal percentage of body fat is in the range of 20 to 25 percent in females, but anorexics often have as little as 5 to 7 percent body fat. Because of the loss of subcutaneous fat, the veins in the skin often seem quite prominent, and the outlines of underlying bones are more visible. (Subcutaneous fat is found just below the skin, so it softens the body contours.) The eyes are sunken, often with a passive look to them. Cheekbones are prominent and the skin of the neck hangs in folds, unsupported by subcutaneous fat. The ribs are easily visible and seem to stand out from the chest—a phenomenon caused by thinning of the muscles and loss of fat between the ribs. The shoulder blades and collarbones are very prominent. Curiously, in some women the fat in the breasts is not lost, so that the shape of the breasts is often fairly well maintained. The weight loss is often most visible in the limbs. Marked muscle wasting produces a frighteningly thin, cadaverous appearance. This muscle wasting is often most apparent in the lower thigh just above the knee.

Decreased Basal Metabolic Rate

"Metabolism" is the word used to describe all of the chemical and physical processes involved in the production of energy within the body. The metabolic rate is a measure of how active and efficient the body is in producing energy, at rest or at work. Someone with a high metabolic rate burns up energy—and blood glucose—faster than someone with a low metabolic rate.

In anorexia nervosa the resting (or basal) metabolic rate is decreased as a result of the starvation. Essentially, the body is trying to conserve energy by making its process of handling energy more efficient—turning down the body's "thermostat" to conserve energy during a time of decreased energy supply. Many body processes (such as the menstrual cycle) either shut down completely or are less active as an adaptation to the decrease. Even body temperature decreases, as the body attempts to conserve energy and heat. The decrease may be slight—only a fraction of a degree—but sometimes it is quite marked. Normal body temperature is 98° Fahrenheit (37° Celsius); in people with anorexia nervosa, temperatures lower than 95° Fahrenheit (35° Celsius) have been measured. This makes the anorexic feel cool all the time, and this lower temperature, combined with the lack of insulation due to loss of subcutaneous fat, makes her unable to tolerate cold. The skin feels cool to the touch, particularly on the limbs, where the blood supply is less. The skin may appear bluish on the hands and feet, because more oxygen than usual is taken from the blood in an effort to use the body's resources more efficiently.

Both heart rate and blood pressure are lowered as the body tries to increase energy conservation. Sometimes these circulatory changes can be striking. The normal heart rate is from 70 to 80 beats per minute, but in someone with anorexia nervosa a pulse of 40 beats a minute is not unusual, and pulses below 30 beats per minute occur. This slow heart rate results in lowered blood pressure, which can cause fainting spells and dizziness, especially when the anorexic stands up after sitting or lying down for some time. Normally, when you stand up, gravity makes blood pool in your legs, and your blood vessels contract to maintain blood pressure. In people with anorexia nervosa this reflex mechanism is impaired, and many anorexics feel lightheaded, or may actually faint, if they change positions quickly.

Changes in the Skin and Hair

Anorexics' skin is often dry, not as pliant as usual, and it may feel rougher. This probably results from the changing metabolism of the skin and the lack of water in the skin cells. The skin often has a light yellow, sallow appearance that makes the anorexic look unwell. In some cases the skin is an orangey-yellow color, because anorexics eat too many vegetables containing carotene (such as squash and carrots). Carotene is an orange-yellow vegetable pigment, and too much of the chemical can actually stain the skin.

Hair changes are seen in everyone with anorexia nervosa. There is increased loss of scalp hair. At any time all of us are losing a certain percentage of hair, perhaps as much as 7 percent, but the loss is balanced by new hair growing in. In anorexics the percentage of hair being lost increases dramatically, up to 25 percent. This excessive hair loss can be easily seen after brushing or combing the hair, and leads to a generalized thinning of the hair. In addition, each hair becomes more fragile, brittle and easily damaged. The hair loses its luster and often the color fades.

Fine, downlike hairs called *lanugo* (from the Latin *lana*, wool) form on the rest of the body and can be quite easily seen on the face, arms and torso. Lanugo is normally seen in newborn infants, but it disappears after the first few months of life. The development of lanugo may result from the body's effort to conserve heat. The fine hairs are thought to trap air close to the body and thus act as a form of insulation.

Loss of Menstrual Cycle

In order to be diagnosed as having anorexia nervosa, a woman of menstruating age must have had amenorrhea for three consecutive months or more. In anorexia nervosa the level of hormones secreted by the brain to activate the ovaries' secretion of hormones is lowered, and so the ovaries do not produce normal levels of the female hormones estrogen and progesterone, and this causes the periods to cease. It's as if the brain has directed that there should be no ovarian function (and therefore no possibility of pregnancy) in such a condition of starvation.

The decrease in body fat is also an important factor in shutting down the brain's ovarian-stimulating hormones. Indeed, the percentage of body fat appears to be much more important in this shutting down than the total body weight. The critical amount of body fat in women in this regard seems to be about 12 percent—below this figure the brain will not stimulate the ovaries into action. In addition, emotional stress by itself has been known to markedly decrease these hormones, and thus the menstrual cycle, even without significant weight loss.

Because the ovaries are inactive in amenorrhea, the body has low levels of female hormones, and what little estrogen and progesterone may be present do not increase and decrease through the month as in normal women. Estrogen is responsible for many secondary sex characteristics—for example, the depositing of fat on the thighs, hips and breasts; the pattern of hair distribution; the maintenance of libido (sexual desire), and so on. Estrogen also plays an important part in the metabolism of calcium in the female skeleton. Low levels of estrogen produce a marked loss of calcium in the bones, a condition called osteoporosis. Bones affected by osteoporosis are more easily broken or crushed.

Insomnia

Most anorexics have sleep difficulties. In particular, they have difficulty falling asleep and have multiple wakenings, and their sleep is much less refreshing. Their total time asleep decreases. They often need naps. Researchers feel that the pursuit of thinness damages the normal restorative function of sleep by preventing the mental relaxation that is necessary for normal sleep.

Excessive Physical Activity

In spite of their dangerous weight loss and obvious loss of muscle mass, most anorexics are very active. Many see a rigorous daily exercise program as part of their pursuit of thinness. They seem to be "addicted" to exercise, seeing it more as a duty than as a pleasure. Even when not exercising, many anorexics are filled with energy—flitting about the room and unable to sit still for long periods of time. In animal studies, starvation is almost always accompanied by an increase in physical activity. This may be a compensating mechanism: the starvation may stimulate more physical activity so that the animal can find more food to solve the starvation problem.

Mental Changes

Many anorexics complain of decreased ability to concentrate and slowness of thinking. There may be less mental activity even though there is more physical activity. Anorexics often fixate on food, and spend much of their time preparing menus, dreaming of food and cooking for others. Depression and social withdrawal are both very common, as is mild confusion. Obsessive-compulsive traits are common. The anorexic characteristically is not concerned about the degree of her weight loss or obvious muscle wasting, but seems indifferent to the severity of the problem. Anorexics often seem to be distant emotionally, hard to reach (even to family members or loved ones), apathetic, uninvolved and aloof.

Fluid Retention

As a result of the altered metabolism caused by starvation, some plasma and other fluids leak out of capillaries (small blood vessels) and cause visible swelling. This is usually notice-

Anorexia nervosa in athletes

Thinness and low body fat are an advantage in some sports that require grace and strength, but in which a particular body shape is expected or approved. Gymnastics, for example, requires incredible strength, agility and flexibility, yet the sport is associated with the image of a childlike body, with very little development of such secondary sexual characteristics as breasts or significant body fat deposits on thighs or buttocks.

Anorexia nervosa is much more common in such sports. In one study of gymnasts, 62 percent were using at least one abnormal form of weight control, such as self-induced vomiting, diet pills, fasting, laxatives or diuretics. (Diuretics cause the body to excrete more water in urine, which lowers body weight.) In the same study it was found that coaches had told two-thirds of female gymnasts that they were "too heavy." Anorexia nervosa is estimated to be 25 times more common in young female gymnasts than it is in the general population. Female figure skaters also show a great drive for thinness, and anorexia nervosa is very common in this group as well.

Dancing, especially ballet, demands a thin body shape coupled with strength and agility. In one study, more than 25 percent of female ballet students aged 11 to 14 showed evidence of an eating disorder. Other female athletics, such as cheerleading, bodybuilding, swimming, diving and distance running, are all associated with an abnormal concern for thinness.

Male athletes are not exempt from this problem. The sport of wrestling causes them the most concern about weight, because many wrestlers try to compete in a weight class that is lower than their normal weight. Although they must maintain their strength, they must also keep their weight unnaturally low. This produces an intense focus on thinness, and often inappropriate methods of weight reduction, such as starvation, dietary or fluid restriction, bulimia, excessive use of laxatives or diuretics, and dehydration.

able in the legs, where gravity makes more fluid leak into surrounding tissue. As a result, anorexics often have puffy-looking ankles and feet, and sometimes other visible edema (swelling caused by fluid retention).

The Statistics

Though many young people have eating disorders, full-blown anorexia nervosa is a relatively rare disease. The annual incidence (the number of new cases reported) of anorexia nervosa is 5 to 10 cases per 100,000 population. It is overwhelmingly a disease of young women, and occurs in about 1 percent of adolescent and adult women in Western society; only about 10 percent of cases occur in men. The average age of onset of the illness is 17 years, though it can occur in girls as young as age 6 or 7 and in post-menopausal women. There is some evidence to suggest that the age of onset is steadily decreasing, and that girls are developing the illness earlier in their lives. About 6 percent of young women have some but not all of the characteristics of the illness. By strict medical criteria these young women cannot be diagnosed as having anorexia nervosa, but they share some of the same problems.

Though the illness was first described centuries ago, there has been a significant increase in the number of cases diagnosed over the past 10 to 15 years. Although earlier research seemed to suggest that the disease was more common in women of upper social classes, more recent studies suggest that this observation may no longer be valid, and that the disease affects equal numbers of sufferers in all social classes.

Anorexia nervosa seems to be limited to the more prosperous countries of the world. In the developing world anorexia is virtually unheard of. It seems that in these less privileged societies, extreme weight loss is usually the result of inadequate nutrition, not willful starvation. In Western

Brain damage and eating disorders

Occasionally, full-blown anorexia nervosa, including distorted body image and fear of weight gain, develops in an older person who has never before had this problem, following brain damage. In a few documented cases, this has appeared after brain trauma such as injury in a car accident. There are also reports of it appearing in someone with a dementia such as Alzheimer's disease. Has the brain damage caused or triggered the eating disorder, or is this just a coincidence? The answer is not yet clear.

countries, the act of voluntarily limiting food intake amid a plentiful supply of food allows the anorexic to demonstrate her control. In some societies, thinness is not nearly as admired as it is in ours. In these countries, dieting to lose weight is not as common a social phenomenon, and anorexia nervosa is less frequent.

Students and other young people who travel from less privileged societies to the West have a much higher incidence of anorexia nervosa than the classmates they leave behind. It seems that the social milieu of the more prosperous country is responsible for the increased incidence of the disease. In newly developed countries such as Korea and Japan, eating disorders are rampant. Even China, where only a few years ago anorexia nervosa was very rarely seen, now has a severe problem with it in major centers.

TWO

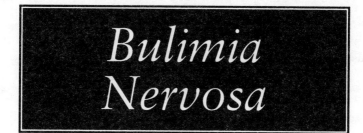

*Bulimia
Nervosa*

Monica awakens to the sound of her morning alarm. She feels tired and her throat is still sore as she gets out of bed to face another day. She's determined that this day will be different.

She gets dressed, makes herself a quick coffee (black, of course) and brushes her teeth for the tenth time in 24 hours. She tells her mother that she doesn't have time to have a regular breakfast this morning, but promises to grab something to eat when she gets to school. She kisses her mom goodbye at the side door, then hops on her bike and rides furiously across town to her first morning class at university. Between classes she grabs another coffee and chews gum to appease her growing hunger. Noon arrives and she allows herself to have lunch, like everyone else, but Monica has only a diet cola and an apple. She feels that she is in control of her problem.

On the way home from school, she stops in at a convenience store and buys a large bag of licorice, a gallon (over four liters) of butterscotch ice cream and two bags of chocolate chip cookies. She pedals home quickly, arriving at four o'clock. She is alone, and knows she will be for at least an hour. She sits in her bedroom and mechanically begins to eat everything she has just purchased. During her binge she leaves her room several times to vomit. The vomiting comes easily. She no longer needs to put her fingers into her mouth—she just thinks about vomiting and she can make it happen.

Now Monica begins to cry again. The familiar, unbearable guilt of bingeing—along with her overwhelming fear of becoming fat, and the horrible stomach pain from gorging—faithfully triggers her need to vomit into the toilet time and time again. After finishing her last morsel and vomiting for the final time, she quickly cleans up the telltale evidence of empty bags, containers of food and dirty dishes. This is her secret. No one must know. She opens the window to the bathroom, sprays the room with air freshener and wipes traces of vomit from the toilet bowl to hide the evidence of her most recent purge. On her hands and knees, cleaning up the vomitus, she feels tired and sad. Today is no different. She is not in control at all.

Monica's mother, father and brother eventually arrive home. They're concerned about her and they know something's not right, but she answers with "I'm all right" though she knows she isn't. How can she tell them? At six p.m. she doesn't sit at the dining-room table for dinner. She excuses her non-participation by stating that she must go to basketball practice immediately. At her mother's insistence, she promises to eat later. "A full meal—just leave it out for me and I'll warm it up." She takes her mother's car and leaves for a basketball practice that does not exist. Instead, Monica goes to the gym to try to lose herself in exercise. She uses the stationary bike for half an hour, lifts weights for another half-hour and does heavy aerobic exercises for another hour and a half. There is no joy in her exercise, only desperation, as if the activity were a punishment. She returns home in the evening and goes straight to her room, after carefully throwing out the plateful of food her mother has left on the kitchen counter. Before bed she does a hundred sit-ups, lifts some more weights and runs on the spot for another 45 minutes. Finally, she allows herself to go to bed. After the rest of the family is asleep, she silently returns to the kitchen at 2:30 a.m. and binges and vomits repeatedly for another two hours.

Monica goes back to her bedroom for the last time this night. The blood she has seen in the toilet bowl and the sharp chest pains she feels from vomiting earlier in the day scare her, and she vows that she will never binge and vomit again. She is sad and frightened. She knows she is out of control. Lying in bed, looking out the bedroom window, she is determined to change her life once and for all.

Monica wakens to her alarm the next morning, only to begin another day in her secret world of bulimia.

The Diagnosis

Bulimia nervosa, more commonly just called bulimia, has only recently been officially classified as an eating disorder. Although it has many similarities to anorexia nervosa, unique properties define it as a distinct eating disorder.

Bulimia nervosa is characterized by two particular behaviors: binge eating, a specific kind of overeating, and purging, the act of trying to rid the body of unwanted food or calories. The word "purge" comes from the Latin *purgare*, to cleanse. Purging behaviors include self-induced vomiting (done in the hope of eliminating recently eaten food) and the use of laxatives, diuretics and rectal suppositories or enemas. Other weight-losing behaviors, such as the use of appetite suppressants and excessive exercising, may be used as well. Purging and over-exercising are often referred to as compensating behaviors, as they are meant to prevent weight gain by compensating for the bingeing.

Medical criteria for the diagnosis of bulimia nervosa

- repeated episodes of binge eating. Binge eating includes both the act of eating excessive amounts of food and the feeling of being unable to stop eating or to limit how much is eaten during the binge
- some sort of behavior to try to lose the weight gained during the binge. These behaviors include such things as vomiting, laxative use, fasting or excessive exercise
- an abnormal feeling that body weight is very important for self-esteem
- repetition of the binge eating and the behaviors at least twice a week for a minimum of three months

Bulimia nervosa is further classified into two subgroups, depending on how the person tries to avoid weight gain. One is called the "purging type"; the person has regularly induced vomiting or misused laxatives, diuretics or enemas. The other is called the "nonpurging type"; the person has used other inappropriate compensating behaviors, such as fasting or excessive exercise, but has not regularly induced vomiting or misused laxatives, diuretics or enemas.

Like anorexics, bulimics often fast or starve themselves to cause weight loss or to prevent weight gain. As well, the individual with bulimia places too much importance on body shape or weight in defining self-worth.

Binge Eating (Bingeing)

An episode of binge eating is medically defined as eating within a specific period of time (for example, within any two-hour period) an amount of food larger than most people would eat, *and* having a sense of lack of control; the bulimic feels she *cannot* stop eating or control what or how much she is eating.

The normal, healthy amount of food that the average adolescent or adult eats daily provides about 1,800 to 2,600 calories. Binge eating may allow a person to eat well over 50,000 calories. This is about 20 to 25 times the normal daily energy intake most of us need to function. As an example, a bulimic may eat two dozen chocolate cookies, two large boxes of cereal and eight pints (over four liters) of ice cream at one sitting. This kind of eating may happen several times a day.

What is hard to define precisely is what a "large" amount of food really is. What is deemed large for one person may be perceived as normal for someone else, and not enough for others. Some experts have tried to define a binge as eating a thousand calories at one sitting, but this is about the caloric content of a hamburger, fries and a cola. Many teenagers consider this just a snack!

Bulimic binges, which may last minutes to an hour or two, usually end in some form of purging, and are usually accompanied by a desperate feeling of being out of control while eating. Bulimics report that they are powerless during the binge. "I can't stop myself once I get started. I numb out and the whole binge is just a blur. I don't even remember what I ate."

Bingeing can happen almost anywhere, any time, and bulimics may overeat voraciously in their homes, at work, at school, in restaurants, in their cars, on the street, or even while shopping, at the beach or in a public park. At home, binges may consist of food already in the cupboards or refrigerator. Some order out for food such as pizza and Chinese food, and binge on this. The bulimic knows the excessive food intake is abnormal, and often goes to great lengths to hide the behavior. For example, it's not uncommon for someone to order two large pizzas by telephone, just for herself, while implying to the person taking the order that she needs food

---

Calories and kilocalories

Although people often talk about the "calories" in food, the scientifically correct term is "kilocalories." There are 1,000 calories in a kilocalorie, or Kcal; the metric equivalent is 4.184 kilojoules.

for a whole group of people. She may even reinforce the illusion by pretending to communicate with others, yelling, "What do you want on your pizza?" to give the person on the other end of the phone the impression that she is ordering for other people.

In their search for a large quantity of food, bulimics may drive around ordering takeout from drive-in fast-food restaurants, one after the other. Convenience stores, where snack foods are plentiful, may be included in such a binge cruise. The bulimic will even drive to distant parts of the city to prevent anyone noticing that she makes frequent visits to convenience stores or restaurants all in one day.

At home, in a dormitory or at the workplace, some bulimics binge on food that does not belong to them. Naturally, this creates suspicion and resentment in family members, co-workers and roommates. Someone working in a restaurant may steal food from the kitchen, buffet, salad bar or even directly from the customers' plates. People may "graze" all day at work, consuming huge quantities of food, unnoticed by fellow employees. Some desperate individuals even rummage in garbage cans for discarded food, while others steal food from the family cat or dog. Some eat their own vomitus when food is not available.

Binges can occur at any time of the day or night. Bulimics often hoard food and keep it hidden away so they can binge secretly and in private late at night, or when others in the house are out.

Bulimics binge on many different types of food, but they often choose items that are denied during periods of dieting or restricting: "junk food," "snack food" or anything high in sugar and fat. These foods are often deliciously sweet or salty, precooked and prepackaged, relatively cheap and available almost anywhere. But any food may be used.

Because of the excessive quantity of food involved, binge-ing can be an extremely expensive behavior. Some bulimics incur little in the way of personal expense because they binge infrequently or binge on other people's food, but others find they are spending several hundred dollars daily on food. This rivals the financial cost of a narcotic addiction. When money is not available for food, some will binge on food received from food banks.

Oddly enough, many bulimics feel that they are bingeing even when they are not truly doing so. They are experiencing a *subjective* binge, a personal feeling that a binge has occurred. In fact, they may have consumed only a normal meal, or even a very small snack. Two soda crackers may seem like a binge to someone who is not psychologically prepared to eat anything. Psychological binges are not real binges, but they demonstrate the sense of lack of control that is characteristic of bulimia.

Purging Behaviors

Purging behaviors are used to eliminate the unwanted food eaten during a binge, and to prevent weight gain. The bulimic succumbs to the overwhelming desire to eat excessively during a binge, and later is filled with remorse and tries to keep the body from absorbing the food. The most common form of purging is vomiting, but misuse of laxatives, diuretics, sup-positories and enemas may also be employed.

Vomiting

Vomiting is used as an attempt to completely empty the stomach during or after a binge, or even after eating normal amounts of food or drink. The vomiting is usually voluntary. Many bulimics use their fingers or some object to tickle the back of the throat (oropharynx). This stimulates the so-called gag reflex, a protective physiological response, and triggers vomiting. Vomiting often becomes easier with practice, and many bulimics learn to vomit at will. When, as sometimes happens, vomiting becomes harder to do, they may panic and go to extremes. They may stand upside down or drink toxic substances to make themselves sick. Very dangerous chemicals, such as liquid dish soap or other cleaning agents, have been used. Some bulimics overdose on drugs, or tell people they have overdosed even though they have not, just to have their stomachs pumped in the hospital emergency room.

Those having difficulty vomiting often use other eating-disorder behaviors, such as restricting (severe dieting) and excessive exercising. Sometimes, bulimics get so used to vomiting that they can no longer control being sick and will vomit at the slightest stimulus, when they least expect it; vomiting becomes, in itself, an involuntary eating-disorder behavior. Some bulimics vomit so easily that they are sick against their will, in front of others at home, in restaurants, at school, in the workplace or at parties with friends, which creates a very embarrassing situation. Some wake up from sleeping and involuntarily vomit onto their bedclothes. This can lead to choking on vomit, which can be fatal if they don't manage to clear the vomitus from their lungs and airway.

Although vomiting can be done almost anywhere there is a drain or toilet bowl, bulimics are ashamed of their vomiting and go to great lengths to hide it. Some vomit into bags or napkins and hide them under the bed, in closets, in cupboards, behind furniture or even in clothing. Often these bags are detected, because the odor of vomitus is very distinctive. Vomiters may use an air freshener to hide the smell, and chew gum or suck on breath mints to mask the smell of vomit on their breath. They may carry a toothbrush to use faithfully after each vomiting session. Some bulimics vomit down the shower drain while taking a shower, hoping others will not be suspicious. Sometimes this clogs the drains, and the plumber discovers that pieces of partially digested food have caused the obstruction.

Digestive tract

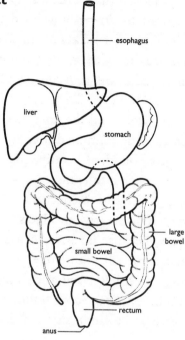

Laxatives

Laxatives are chemicals that stimulate the bowel to help evacuate stool (feces) from the body. They are available in pill, capsule or liquid form. Some of these chemicals are relatively safe while others are very dangerous.

Bulimics use laxatives in the hope that food eaten during a binge will be rushed out of the stomach and through the intestines before a significant amount of nutrition can be absorbed. This is a false belief. Nutrition from food is absorbed in the small bowel, which, on average, is 20 feet (6 m) long. The small bowel is so efficient at absorbing nutrients that most nutrition is absorbed no matter how quickly the food travels through it. But laxatives work mainly in the large bowel, where nutrient absorption does not occur; the large bowel functions only to remove water from the semi-liquid waste. Thus laxatives do not usually affect the absorption of calories. Typically, the only weight lost is that of the water that is evacuated. Many laxatives irritate the lower bowel and cause an abnormal secretion of liquid, which makes up much of the diarrhea.

When laxatives are first used, a small amount can work to increase the number of bowel movements. One pill a day is all most people need. However, the body soon develops a tolerance to these chemicals, and the dose needed to stimulate the bowel increases with continued use. Some bulimics use two hundred or three hundred laxative pills a day, because they have developed such a tolerance.

Bulimics take great lengths to conceal any evidence of laxative misuse. Some hide laxative products in cigarette packages or in drawers. Because laxatives cause diarrhea, there may be a telltale residue left in the toilet bowl, as well as an odor, so cleaning the toilet bowl and using air freshener become a common practice. Some bulimics even defecate down the shower drain to hide signs of diarrhea resulting from laxative abuse.

Laxatives can cause excessive fluid loss and result in chemical disruption in the body (see below). These medications are also expensive, especially if they are used regularly and in large quantities. They can cost hundreds of dollars yearly.

Diuretics (Water Pills)

Diuretics are chemicals that cause a person to produce more urine than usual. Normally, the kidneys regulate the volume of urine produced, and the balance of waste chemicals dissolved in urine that the body needs to eliminate at any given time. This is an important function of the kidneys, which quickly adjust the volume and chemical concentrations of the urine to maintain the correct balance for proper health. Diuretics cause weight loss by removing only water from the body; they have no effect on removing fat or calories. Most diuretics are prescription drugs, although some over-the-counter versions are found in health food stores. Diuretics commonly produce dehydration because of excessive loss of body fluid through urine, and disruption of body chemicals.

Suppositories

Rectal suppositories are solid, elongated objects that are inserted through the anus into the rectum with the purpose of evacuating feces from the bowel. Suppositories contain chemicals that irritate the lower bowel and thus cause reflex emptying. Bulimics use suppositories thinking that they will lose weight. Rectal suppositories have *no effect* on preventing food from being absorbed or on getting rid of fat from the body.

Enemas

An enema is a liquid preparation instilled into the lower bowel to cause evacuation of the bowel. Enemas work similarly to rectal suppositories, by irritating the bowel. They are inserted through the anus with an applicator. Like laxatives, they can be expensive and habit-forming.

Bulimia Nervosa: A Newly Recognized Disorder?

The concept of extreme overeating is not new. For over two millennia, descriptions of overeating or of eating an excessive quantity of food in a voracious or hurried manner have been frequent. As the word "anorexia" means a lack of hunger, bulimia has been thought of as hyperorexia ("hyper" meaning excessive), or a heightened, exaggerated hunger.

The word "bulimia" is derived from the Greek *bous*, "ox," and *limos*, "hunger," and may imply that someone possesses an appetite as big as an ox's, or has the capability of eating a whole ox. Bulimia has been identified by many different names. It has been called *boolmot* (Hebrew), *bulimy* (Greek), morbid hunger, phegedaena, hound's appetite, canine appetite, bolilsmus, bolimos, cynorexia, *Ess Sucht* (German "craving for eating") and gluttony.

Deliberate vomiting also has a history dating back to ancient times. We have all heard stories of the Romans eating and then inducing vomiting so that they could eat some more. Seneca, a Roman philosopher and statesman, is quoted as saying, "Men eat to vomit and vomit to eat." The ancient Egyptians would consume substances (called emetics) to make them vomit for a few days each month, to prevent disease that they attributed to food. Morbid hunger, which was described in the fifth century, did not just mean to overeat, but was characterized by a ravenous appetite, absence of chewing, and vomiting. Saint Catherine of Siena, who lived in the fourteenth century, starved herself for very long periods of time as a form of spiritual fulfillment. When she did eat, she forced herself to vomit as a punishment for breaking her sacred vow to not eat. She eventually starved to death. In the nineteenth century, *bulimia emetica* was the term for vomiting after eating a large quantity of food.

As well as vomiting, people in the sixth century would deliberately infest their intestines with worms after overeating. Once in the system, the worms prevented the absorption of the excess food.

In the nineteenth century, voracious eating was attributed to medical causes such as head injury, brain disease, hydrocephalus and epilepsy.

Bulimia nervosa was first defined as a specific set of behaviors by Dr. Gerald Russell, a psychiatrist who worked at the Royal Free Hospital in London, England, in 1979. He deter-

Were the Roman emperors bulimic?

In the politically stable and very prosperous early years of the Roman Empire it was common practice to enjoy food to excess. Huge banquets, with large quantities of exotic foods gathered from distant parts of the empire, were served as symbols of wealth and power to a pampered elite. At the time, some of the most famous physicians of antiquity, including Hippocrates, recommended the use of emetics as an intermittent cleansing measure, and these agents were often used to induce vomiting after excessive eating so that guests could return to the banquet table.

According to the historian Petronius, the Roman emperor Claudius "left the dining room bloated and sodden, then, when asleep, had his servants insert a feather into his throat to induce vomiting to relieve his stomach." Emperor Vitellius was a huge man, given to disgusting gluttony and frequent binge eating as well as habitual vomiting through expensive banquets with combination of rare foods such as peacock brains and flamingo tongues. He had such a ravenous appetite that, according to Suetonius' *The Lives of the Caesars*, he also "snatched the sacrificial cakes from the church altar or ate the previous day's half-eaten scraps." Both men drank to excess, though neither seems to have had one of the essential components of bulimia nervosa—a morbid fear of fatness. There was even a special room—the vomitorium—where people could swallow their emetics so that the sound and smell of the vomiting would not interfere with the sensual pleasures of the other guests.

mined that the three criteria for a diagnosis of bulimia nervosa were episodic overeating, vomiting and/or laxative abuse and a fear of fatness. Considerable time has been spent by researchers trying to find evidence that bulimia nervosa was recognized long before 1979. However, very few cases of this syndrome are fully documented before this time. It seems that bulimia nervosa has only recently been identified as a disorder in itself.

Medical Consequences of Bulimia Nervosa

People who engage in bulimic behaviors experience various physical changes. The changes they feel within their bodies are called symptoms, and those that may be observed by others are called signs. Many of these physical alterations may indicate impending health risks. Unfortunately, all too often there are no specific physical signs or symptoms to warn the person of serious or even catastrophic medical problems.

Physical Changes from Repeated Vomiting

The act of vomiting may lead to various physical changes and health risks. People often complain of a sore throat after vomiting. This is often due to the acidic stomach contents passing through the throat, but the pain may also result from scratches left on the roof of the mouth or throat by fingernails, when people use their fingers to induce vomiting. Vomiting can cause painful cracks in the corners of the mouth (cheilosis). Sometimes the force of repeated vomiting can cause broken blood vessels to appear around the eyes, or even cause bleeding on the surface of the eyes.

The teeth and gums may show permanent damage. Dentists can identify bulimics by tooth damage and a characteristic pattern of inflammation of the gums. Tooth enamel often erodes due to the acids in the vomit, and brushing the teeth soon after vomiting may cause further erosion of the enamel. The gums may recede, especially from repeated harsh brushing. It is not uncommon for vomiters to require caps on their teeth, or oral surgery to repair receding gums. These last two procedures cost many thousands of dollars, and some people with bulimia nervosa need to have dental caps and gum repairs done more than once, if they do not stop vomiting.

Scars created by the teeth rubbing on the top of the hand during forceful thrusting of the hand to the back of the mouth are called Russell's sign, after Dr. Gerald Russell, who first described it. One of the most noticeable physical signs of someone who vomits is the swelling of the salivary glands— most obviously the parotid glands, located immediately in front of and below each ear. When they are swollen, the vomiter's face suggests that of a chipmunk. Sometimes the swelling will go away after vomiting behaviors have stopped, but often the glands remain permanently swollen.

Esophagus

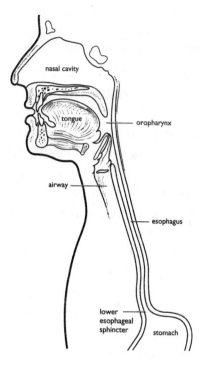

Frequent vomiting may lead to a weakening of the lower esophageal sphincter, a circular area of muscle located at the lower end of the esophagus and designed to prevent stomach contents from entering the esophagus. This weakening allows acidic stomach contents to flow backward into the esophagus at any time, but especially when you are lying down. Someone with this problem, called *reflux*, notices a gnawing or heartburn sensation in the mid-chest as acid from the stomach comes up into the esophagus, irritating the thin mucous lining. There may also be an acidic, irritated feeling in the throat from reflux, and even a sour or bitter taste from the acid. Some people develop chronic sore throats from reflux activity. Ulcers can develop in the esophagus, and these may lead to scarring. This narrows the esophagus, leading to difficulty in swallowing as food is blocked from entering the stomach. This may necessitate surgery to release the scar tissue and allow food to pass through.

Forceful or repeated vomiting may create very dangerous complications, including the formation of small tears in the lining of the esophagus (Mallory-Weiss tears) or even the complete bursting or rupture of the esophagus. When the esophagus bursts open, air and stomach contents enter the space surrounding the heart and between the lungs, causing life-threatening complications. The stomach itself can be torn by forceful vomiting episodes, just as it can by binge eating, causing the acidic stomach contents to enter the abdominal cavity. This is an extreme emergency and can be fatal. The vomiter experiences pain during or after vomiting, from tears of the esophagus and stomach; fresh blood, or black, partially digested blood, may appear in vomit or in the toilet-bowl water. Anyone who notices chest pain and blood while vomiting must *seek medical attention immediately*.

Bleeding from irritation or smaller tears in the stomach or esophagus may not be immediately noticeable, but can lead to dizziness, weakness and fainting due to anemia—an abnormally low level of red blood cells. Unconsciousness is possible, and even death due to massive internal blood loss. If the stools are black blood loss will be suspected, since the iron from red blood cells turns black in the bowel from partial digestion within the intestine.

Vomiters can also die from vomit or food that is inhaled accidentally during bingeing and vomiting. The vomit or food trapped in the airways of the lungs causes suffocation.

Vomiting may lead to significant health risks involving other organs of the body. The heart and kidneys are put at great risk from dehydration and electrolyte disturbances created by vomiting, especially in combination with the use of laxatives and diuretics. Electrolytes are chemicals that every cell in the body requires to function—including cells of the heart, brain and kidneys. Disturbances in essential chemicals such as sodium, chloride, potassium, bicarbonate, urea, creatinine and phosphorus can lead to heart problems, including heart rhythm dysfunction that can result in sudden death.

Physical Effects of Binge Eating
Binge eating itself is often associated with physical symptoms. People feel bloated or "stuffed" after overeating. They get

Vomiting and diarrhea as medical treatments
Since antiquity, physicians have prescribed emetics to induce vomiting as a means of purification and treatment of disease. Ancient Egyptians purged themselves by making themselves vomit for three days each month, using cow's milk or infusions of fennel (a parsley-like herb) and honey to empty the stomach, because they believed that "all diseases which men are subject to proceed from the food itself."

In ancient Greece, Hippocrates advised vomiting for two consecutive days per month, reasoning that "ailments caused by excessive fullness are best treated by evacuation." In ancient Arabia, Avicenna recommended vomiting if one "ate to excess," suggesting the use of a finger or feather, assisted by "any gentle laxative such as the confection of roses." However, he warned of the danger of the practice; "to procure vomiting to an undue degree is injurious for the stomach, and is also prejudicial to the thorax and to the teeth."

This practice of trying to eliminate spoiled food or other contaminants that would cause disease continued into the Middle Ages in Europe, by which time cathartic drugs (those that produce diarrhea) became more popular. Mercury was used to rapidly and forcibly empty the bowel of disease, and by the seventeenth century a combination of vomiting and diarrhea was the commonest form of medical therapy for many illnesses—in a desperate and mistaken attempt to rid the body of the agents that caused disease.

We now understand that vomiting and diarrhea are not effective treatments of disease at all. Instead, they weaken the body through loss of fluid and other essential chemicals, and they are never prescribed.

abdominal cramps and pains due to the large amount of food rapidly distending the stomach. Individuals have been known to overeat to such a degree that the stomach actually ruptures from massive stretching. This produces sudden, severe pain in the abdomen and is a medical emergency.

Problems from Misusing Laxatives

Laxative abuse can lead to several physical symptoms other than diarrhea. Laxatives cause mild to severe bowel cramps as they overstimulate the gut to create bowel movements. They can cause nausea. Pain in the area of the anus develops as a result of frequent diarrhea and wiping after bowel movements. Discontinuing laxatives abruptly can cause constipation and bloating because the large bowel has adapted to the artificial stimulation and will not function easily on its own; a doctor viewing the bowel with a sigmoidoscope may not see a normal, pale pink color, but a black color caused by the overuse of laxatives. Prolonged use of laxatives can actually poison the nerve network of the bowel, so that it no longer functions. This may require surgical removal of the affected part of the bowel to allow proper functioning. Laxatives can also lead to falling, fainting or even death as a result of dehydration and electrolyte disturbances similar to those created by vomiting.

Problems from Misusing Diuretics

By interfering with the kidneys' regulatory effects on fluid and body chemical balance, diuretics cause excessive and inappropriate loss of fluid from the body—fluid that contains essential elements such as electrolytes. This combination produces dehydration and chemical imbalance, which in turn causes thirst, dizziness, low blood pressure, fatigue, muscle cramping and fainting.

Problems from Over-exercising

Exercise is an essential activity for health, but it is often used to excess by bulimics as a method of controlling weight or hunger, or as a form of self-punishment. Exercise in excess can lead to numerous ailments and health risks. The most common physical complaints are aches and pains of the lower limbs and back from repetitive exercise regimes such as running and sit-ups. Joint pains, swelling and stiffness may develop in ankles, knees and hips from running, jogging and power-walking. Stress fractures of the bones in the feet and shins may develop from frequent, repeated hard exercise of the lower limbs. Exercise only aggravates the back pains associated with the thinning bones of osteoporosis. Exercise-induced injuries can cause someone with an eating disorder to panic, because these injuries can limit or totally prevent daily exercising and thus diminish her ability to control her weight. Fear of weight gain because of a lack of exercise may prime an individual to put increased effort into other bulimic behaviors, such as vomiting.

The more you are exposed to street physical activities such as running or cycling, the more you are at risk of being hit by vehicles, as well as experiencing typical sport-related injuries such as spraining an ankle. The sometimes preoccupied mind of the frantic exerciser, who is focused on losing weight, puts her at particular risk of such accidents. Some such people become accident-prone, experiencing a series of exercise-induced injuries.

Problems from Misusing Emetics

Emetics are chemicals that are swallowed to produce vomiting. Some emetics are very dangerous and may cause death. Emetine, a chemical found in one commercial emetic, becomes stored in muscle tissue after repeated use. It builds up toxic levels in muscles and results in weakness of the skeletal muscles found in the arms and legs and the chest wall. The heart, being made up of muscle tissue, becomes poisoned as well, and this can lead to complete heart failure and death. Two doses of emetine a week can cause death in some individuals, after a period of time.

Emetics can produce such violent vomiting that stomach and esophageal tears become more likely. Massive hemorrhages (bleeding) from these tears, or actual rupturing of the stomach or esophagus, will most certainly lead to death.

Statistics

Statistics for bulimia nervosa have only been kept since about 1980. Precise figures are impossible to establish since most published reports come from hospital and university centers, where only a small proportion of the bulimic population has been observed. Because bulimia is often a secret disorder, the bulimic makes great attempts to hide her behavior from family and professionals. The few statistics that are available are from developed countries, not from developing ones.

Some studies report the average occurrence of bulimia nervosa as one in a hundred. Approximately 90 percent to 95 percent of those with bulimia nervosa are female. Male bulimics are often harder to identify because they seem to avoid seeking help from caregivers even more often than females. The incidence of bulimic symptoms, based on surveys using questionnaires, has been determined to be as high as 19 percent among female students.

Bulimia nervosa most commonly begins during or after puberty, and very rarely before puberty, but can be seen at any age. In one study, the mean age of onset of bulimia nervosa was 13.9 years old, with a range of 11 to 15 years as the age when the disorder first appeared.

Many people with bulimia successfully hide their problem from others, even their doctors. In studies in England and Holland, general practitioners were able to accurately identify 40 percent of their patients who had anorexia nervosa, but only 11 percent of those who suffered from bulimia. People with bulimia are harder to identify because they often do not develop the emaciated body of the anorexic. They may be overweight, underweight or normal. It is interesting to note that 79 percent of those diagnosed with anorexia nervosa are referred on for mental health care, while only 51 percent of those with bulimia are referred on.

THREE

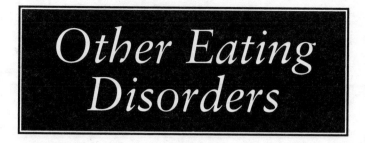

Other Eating Disorders

The more clinicians and researchers learn about eating disorders, the more they realize that these disorders are on a continuum of disordered eating. Anorexia nervosa and bulimia nervosa are only two specific eating disorders out of many. Also, within each of these specific disorders there is another continuum, a wide variation of behavior and attitude from person to person.

Is It a "True" Eating Disorder or a Form of Disordered Eating?

Anorexia nervosa, bulimia nervosa and binge-eating disorder have become accepted as the "true" eating disorders, well defined and studied. Most other kinds of disordered eating that are not direct variations of these three are not considered true "eating disorders." One reason is that other disordered-eating illnesses are not yet well described and studied, and need further investigation. Another reason is that, for someone to be diagnosed with anorexia nervosa or bulimia, there must be an inordinate and abnormal focus on weight or body-image control. If there is no significant unhealthy focus on weight or body image, people with starvation, bingeing or purging behaviors are considered, by definition, not to

Leptin: the hormone of obesity?

The relationship between the type and amount of food we eat, our total weight and percentage of fat and the energy we expend is a complex physiological system that is not completely understood.

In 1994 a new hormone, produced by fat cells and involved in the regulation of weight and the feeling of satiety, was discovered and called leptin (from the Greek *leptos*, meaning thin). Leptin is secreted by fat cells (and also, in lesser amounts, by the cells of the lining of the stomach, the placenta and some fetal tissues). Leptin levels are high in obese humans, and dieting lowers these levels. Patients with anorexia nervosa have very low levels of leptin in their bloodstream, but these levels rise to normal quickly when food intake increases to normal levels. Laboratory mice given leptin by injection show a dramatic appetite reduction—in one study, after four days of daily leptin injections the mice ate 60 percent less food.

It appears that leptin has many different effects and influences a range of processes (for example, insulin secretion, the transportation of sugar, the feeling of satiety, certain reproductive functions, etc.), and exerts at least some of these effects on the hypothalamus, the area in the brain responsible for the feeling of satiety. Human obesity may result from insensitivity (resistance) to the hormone, or from decreased production of the hormone (about 8 percent of morbidly obese humans have markedly decreased levels of leptin in their blood).

However, leptin's effects, and how the hormone fits into the complicated system of energy expenditure and appetite, are not completely known at this time.

have a true eating disorder. For the sake of convenience the term "true eating disorders" will be used to refer to the three more commonly accepted conditions.

Multiple Variables

If you were to listen to the stories of a hundred individuals with anorexia nervosa and a hundred individuals with bulimia, they would all be different. Many different types of eating-disorder attitudes and behaviors can be adopted by any one individual. As well, the intensity and frequency of each behavior or attitude varies. One person with bulimia binges and diets while another binges, vomits and uses laxatives, yet both are diagnosed with bulimia. Some have severe weight-control issues while others don't.

Some people develop eating disorders at a very young age, while others do not develop obvious eating-disorder attitudes and behaviors until very late in life. Some recover at an earlier age than others.

Hunger and fullness signals vary from one person to another. Some people feel normal hunger and fullness. Some experience ravenous hunger while others describe having no hunger signals at all. Some feel full after eating very small amounts of food; others feel they are never full.

Other variables include the comfort with which you live with an eating disorder, your motivation to recover, your weight and rate of weight change and your medical risks.

Given the number of variables and the infinite individual approaches to these variables, it's no wonder there is confusion about identifying the kind of eating disorder someone has, and monitoring the evolution of the disorder, and the recovery.

The Spectrum of Body Image and Weight Control

Western society has a wide range of awareness of body image and weight concern. Some people have no significant concerns and are comfortable with their bodies. Others have a pathological concern with their weight and give up all life's opportunities just to maintain a low weight or to lose weight. Most of us are somewhere between these two extremes.

Similarly, there are those who suffer from disordered eating but have no significant body-image issues that affect their eating. Some people have weight concerns but their behavior is not specifically affected by these issues. As an example, those who binge eat may feel they would *like* to lose weight, yet may not diet, vomit, take laxatives or over-exercise regularly to control their weight. Some have an accurate view of their body shape while others have a severely distorted body image, seeing themselves as severely overweight when, in fact, they are very underweight.

Most people with anorexia nervosa or bulimia begin one of these true eating disorders with overpowering body-image issues, and then pursue weight loss. Indeed, their severe body-image problem is part of the definition of the disorder. Some, however, lose weight despite having no obvious weight-control issues initially, then drift into stronger body-image control patterns. For example, someone who has lost weight while ill may wish to maintain her new weight after receiving praise for her weight-loss accomplishment. Some people deny that they are trying to control their weight because they truly do not believe that they have any body-image issues; it is not until they are challenged to improve their eating and to give up weight-control behaviors that the underlying body-image feelings come to the surface. As recovery proceeds, the fixation on body image will wane. What was once an all-consuming drive for weight control becomes a much weakened drive, overridden by a stronger desire to recover.

There are also people who have profound concern for their body shape, who are very self-conscious about this, but will not do anything to control their weight. They have the body-image fears, and they may be emotionally traumatized by these concerns, but they have not translated their concerns into weight-loss behaviors.

External and Internal Drives to Control Body Image and Weight
Body-image and weight-control drives have both internal and external sources and forces. Examples of external pressures are those created by the media, our family and friends, or the dance teacher who expects an unrealistically low body weight.

The riddles of disordered eating

"I don't know whether I ever had an eating disorder or not. Some people say I did ... others say I didn't.

"Off and on, for years, I wasn't able to eat anything for periods of time. I sometimes couldn't eat for days. The problem was that, if I didn't know where a certain food came from, I couldn't eat it. If I bought an apple at a market my mind would say, 'Where did the apple come from?' If I didn't know that it came from a particular tree, I couldn't stop thinking about it and I wouldn't eat it. If, however, an apple came from a tree in my back yard, I could eat it without worry. This problem resulted in me losing over 30 pounds, but I never ever wanted to lose weight and I had never dieted. I saw a therapist about this and it became clear that I was dealing with a form of obsessive-compulsive disorder. After being started on a small dose of medication to help control my obsessions and compulsions, I was able to eat anything I wanted to, when I wanted to. As long as I keep taking my medication, I'm all right.

"My daughter had a problem with food too. At 12, she would get stomach cramps and become nauseated after eating or drinking, to the point where she would have to vomit. She would then refuse to eat, just to stop the cramps and nausea. This went on for over five years. She ended up missing several months of school each year. She not only didn't gain weight as she should have during her adolescent years, but actually lost weight. Over the years she was seen by several specialists. She was seen once by an adolescent psychiatrist to help determine whether she had anorexia nervosa, and whether there were any particular psychological stressors in her life that could lead to such behaviors. No diagnosis of anorexia nervosa could be made, and there were no particular emotional issues to drive her condition. She had also been assessed by several pediatricians and gastroenterologists. X-rays of her intestines were performed, as well as two sets of biopsies of her colon and stomach, to rule out bowel disease. Again, nothing could be found. She was twice sent to a specialized children's gastroenterology unit at a university hospital, where she stayed for a few weeks and underwent more tests, all to no avail. After a cyst ruptured on one of her ovaries, she was prescribed the birth control pill to help prevent more cysts from growing. Immediately, all her stomach pains and nausea disappeared. Of course, her vomiting stopped as well. She quickly gained weight and she has never looked back."

Internal pressures are those we all create for ourselves, which may be initiated by these external sources or by what we incorrectly interpret as external pressure. For instance, you may feel that others think you are overweight when in fact they do not. Internal drives to control weight can also emerge on their own.

Internal drives to lose weight can persist after the external influences are long gone. As an example, someone may have been teased about her weight eight years ago, and this may remain a trigger for her to diet severely and to vomit.

Binge-Eating Disorder

Binge-eating disorder is the most recently defined and classified true eating disorder. It is, however, possibly one of the oldest forms of disordered eating, although little is known about it in history.

Binge-eating disorder is best understood as bulimia without regular purging, dieting or excessive exercising. It consists of a pattern of recurring binges without compensating behaviors (such as vomiting) to try to lose the weight that may be gained during the binges.

Dieting is quite common in this disorder, but the dieting regime is likely to be intermittent rather than persistent, and is often not strict. Aside from true binges, those who have binge-eating disorder will often overeat at normal mealtimes. Typical meals are unusually large and snacking is excessive.

Binge-eating disorder is extremely common. It affects men and women almost equally, and there is little variation by cultural background. The disorder affects individuals over a broader age range than bulimia or anorexia typically does. Half the people with this disorder are overweight.

The definition of a binge for binge-eating disorder is the same as that for bulimia nervosa and anorexia nervosa: a binge is the consumption of an inordinate amount of food in a specific period of time during which the consumer feels out of control. Eating is rapid, often at twice the rate at which others eat. Eating may initially bring some pleasure but, overall, food generally gives no pleasure. Food is practically "inhaled." Some people say, "I don't even taste what I'm eating."

Those with binge-eating disorder are more likely not to feel full after excessive eating, and may devour volumes of food that others would be unable to consume. The signals for normal fullness seem to be diminished or absent, whereas the threshold for fullness in those with anorexia nervosa or bulimia is lower. Binge eaters eat large amounts of food when they do not feel physically hungry, and they eat alone due to feelings of embarrassment. They commonly feel guilt, disgust with themselves, and depression.

How Does Normal Overindulging Differ from Bingeing?

The average person overeats from time to time, such as during festive and religious occasions. How is that overeating not part of binge-eating disorder? If overeating or bingeing is not causing you any significant disruption in life, any emotional pain or risk to your health, or is not particularly frequent, it is unlikely that you have binge-eating disorder. Overeating at social functions or during festive holidays is generally considered normal and even expected. These indulgences are usually met with more pleasure than distress.

The health risks from binge-eating disorder are the same as those from bulimia. Tears in the stomach may cause pain and bleeding, and in rare instances cause a fatal rupture of the stomach. Other health risks, such as diabetes, high blood pressure, heart attack and stroke, may increase if obesity results from binge-eating.

Dieting and Binge-Eating Disorder

Many people with binge-eating disorder diet, although not as severely as those with anorexia nervosa or bulimia. Many of

How do people feel about their eating disorders?

"My eating disorder is to do with bingeing (not purging), usually after I've come home with my refill of groceries. I want to sample all the fun or tasty categories, so I start with some of this and some of that. I've done it to such an extent that I'm absolutely stuffed with food and drink, my belly feeling pushed out and me feeling filled up to the top of my throat. It's also to do with nonstop snacking ... starting with something, thinking I'll only have one but returning again and again for yet another, even though I may not be hungry or truly desiring that item. It's just something to satisfy or fill a certain something, that keeps me returning for more."

"It means isolation, loneliness, secrecy, lying, depression, feeling hungry, restrictiveness."

those who binge have dieted in the past; others have been overeating or bingeing for years prior to their first diet. But dieting plays an important role in the initiation and continuation of the disorder. Dieting followed by binge eating followed by dieting to lose the weight gained creates a cycle, since the relative starvation of dieting predisposes the person to another binge. Other weight-losing behaviors, such as vomiting or over-exercising, can perpetuate this cycle. Anorexia nervosa and bulimia can both lead to binge-eating disorder. Obesity, which sometimes precedes binge-eating disorder, may itself trigger binge eating, due to the dieting and other weight-loss behaviors many obese people adopt.

Night Eating Disorder

Binge eating can occur at any time during the day, but excessive food intake at night is fairly common and is seen in two distinct patterns.

In some binge eaters, often as a result of stresses such as family conflicts, relationship breakups and social situations, a distinct pattern of eating develops. These people are not hungry at all in the morning and are only slightly hungry in the afternoon. However, they overeat in the time from supper until midnight or the early hours of the morning. This evening *hyperphagia* (overeating) occurs frequently, two or three times a week, and often consists of consuming an excessive amount of sweet or high-calorie foods.

In addition, these binge eaters suffer from insomnia. They have difficulty getting to sleep and difficulty staying asleep, and an irritable sleeplessness, although they are wide awake when they are eating.

A more bizarre form of night eating disorder occurs in some people: they overeat while sleepwalking. They are actually asleep, usually deeply asleep, when they arise from bed and in an automatic fashion head to the kitchen. In the kitchen they proceed to eat large quantities of food. Sweets and pasta are the preferred foods, but sometimes, in their sleepwalking state, they eat inappropriate items such as uncooked fish sticks, raw bacon, bread covered with sugar, sunflower oil, raw, frozen or spoiled foods, and even buttered cigarettes. Many of these people are inattentive or sloppy with food preparation. Some are injured during careless cutting of food or opening of cans, or while consuming very hot liquids or solids; some run into walls, counters, tables or other objects. After the binge-eating episode, the sleepwalker returns to bed. This may happen repeatedly—up to eight times per night. Not all of the feedings are binges; sometimes only a small amount of food or liquid is taken. There is no purging after the binge, and there are no complaints of abdominal pain, nausea or a feeling of fullness.

Night bingers tend to drink thick fluids (for example, milkshakes) and consume thick foods (especially peanut butter, ice cream and candy bars). Sometimes they eat the food raw or uncooked, but sometimes entire hot or cold meals are prepared.

In the morning, on awakening, they don't recall the specifics of the eating episode, but they find the evidence in the kitchen: empty boxes and food containers and signs of food preparation.

Sleepwalking bingers frequently feel dejected and disgusted in the morning over their loss of control. They often resolve nightly to try to control the pattern of behavior. But because the behavior occurs during sleep, it is impossible for them to control it.

Medication for this type of eating disorder is available: clonazepam, a drug that relieves anxiety, may be effective, and is sometimes combined with fluoxetine (an antidepressant).

Eating Disorders Not Otherwise Specified

The eating disorders defined as "not otherwise specified" (NOS) are all at least partially related to anorexia nervosa or bulimia nervosa.

NOS eating disorders similar to anorexia nervosa are those that fulfill all of the criteria for anorexia nervosa except one. As an example, a 15-year-old girl who has a distorted body image, has not had her period for six months and has lost 11 percent of her total body weight is not classified as having anorexia nervosa because she has not lost 15 percent or more of her healthy weight. A 21-year-old woman who has lost 17 percent of her body weight due to deliberate weight-loss dieting but still has her period is similarly not classified as having anorexia nervosa, but as having an NOS eating disorder. (Some researchers have argued that the presence of a menstrual period should not exclude someone from a diagnosis of anorexia nervosa.)

People with NOS eating disorders related to bulimia are those who binge, purge and have other compensatory behaviors but have the behaviors less often than twice per week. It may be that someone vomits after eating small amounts of food (e.g., two cookies) and not after real binges. Others do

The man in the mirror
Although eating disorders are found mostly among women, men have their own problems with body image. Those with a disorder called *muscle dysmorphia*—sometimes nicknamed "bigorexia" or "reverse anorexia"—see themselves as shamefully weak and puny even if they're bulging with muscles. While anorexic women starve themselves to remove imaginary fat, men with muscle dysmorphia may spend endless hours at the gym; some even quit lucrative and prestigious jobs so that they can work out more. Just as women may be embarrassed to be seen at a beach in a bathing suit for fear of being seen as fat, men will avoid taking their shirt off in public or going to beaches because they feel grossly inadequate as male figures. They may resort to illegal steroids and other drugs that can lead to infertility, high blood pressure, liver failure and death. Men with muscle dysmorphia may also develop anorexia nervosa or bulimia.

not actually binge and purge but they chew large amounts of food and then deliberately spit it out, to avoid weight gain. This is not bulimia by definition, but it is an eating disorder of the NOS group.

Eating Disorders in Children
Children quite commonly develop various forms of disordered eating. Some of these disorders develop due to the conscious desire to lose weight, as with anorexia nervosa or bulimia of childhood, while others develop for different reasons.

Children with Anorexia Nervosa and Bulimia Nervosa
True anorexia nervosa and bulimia are rarely seen in young children. Although very young children may be aware of body image and feel pressure to lose weight, they seldom actively begin to diet to try to control weight until their teen years.

Anorexia nervosa has been identified in children as young as six or seven, although of course prepubertal girls are lacking one usual criterion for defining anorexia: missing three or more periods. For a child to be diagnosed as anorexic, there has to be a history of a morbid fear of becoming fat, just as in adolescents and adults. Bulimia is seldom seen before puberty.

Anorexia nervosa is especially dangerous in younger children because their weight loss represents a loss of more lean body mass than for adolescents or adults. Acute and significant weight loss in children can be life-threatening, and must be treated as a medical emergency.

Pervasive Refusal Syndrome

First described by Dr. Bryan Lask and his colleagues in England in 1991, pervasive refusal syndrome is a very rare condition characterized by dramatic social withdrawal and profound refusal to eat, drink, walk, talk or maintain personal hygiene. Lask originally described instances of four girls from 9 to 14 years of age with these behaviors. One of the girls had developed symptoms of anorexia nervosa prior to her pervasive refusal state, while the others had not.

Since this initial study, pervasive refusal syndrome has been identified in children elsewhere in the world. The reasons proposed for a child adopting such extreme behavior include a history of sexual abuse or some other traumatic experience, including severe family dysfunction, or social deprivation. This syndrome may evolve as a kind of post-traumatic stress disorder. More recently, there is evidence that it may represent a form of learned helplessness—a method of coping with chronic stress by forcing others to make decisions, and to provide desperately needed attention.

Treatment involves both individual and family therapy, with care provided in a hospital. Lengthy hospital stays are usually required.

Selective Eating

Children with selective eating will eat only two or three different foods, and go to great lengths to adamantly refuse other nourishment. These children are typically of normal weight and height, and they do not seem to be eliminating food choices as a way to control weight; fear of weight gain is not an issue. Parents worry that their child is not being adequately nourished. However, most children grow out of this phase before their nutrition is significantly affected.

Appetite Loss Secondary to Depression

Depression affects children in much the same way as it affects adults, but it is often not diagnosed as easily. After selective eating and weight control have been ruled out as causes when a child is unwilling to eat, a medical cause or depression should be suspected. Depressed children refuse to eat because of a genuine loss of appetite (as contrasted with children with anorexia nervosa, who have a normal or even increased appetite but suppress it). Depressed children who lose weight due to a lack of desire to eat are often misdiagnosed with anorexia nervosa, which delays appropriate treatment.

Children who truly suffer from anorexia nervosa, however, often experience depression at the same time as they have their eating disorder. These children have two powerful forces influencing their desire to eat: the desire to lose weight and a true lack of appetite.

Pica

"Pica" is the medical term for a tendency or craving to eat substances that are not fit as food and have no nutritional value. The word *pica* is Latin for "magpie," a bird known for collecting and hoarding bright objects and for its voracious and indiscriminate appetite. Pica has been described for centuries and is fairly common today. Objects eaten include such things as ice chips, coins, cigarette butts, dried paint chips, carpet fiber, flour, clay, chalk, toothpaste, leaves, baking powder, laundry soap, starch, coffee grounds and matches.

Pica is fairly common in pregnancy (one study found that it was present in 20 percent of pregnant women), and is sometimes seen in people with deficiencies of iron and zinc, disappearing once the deficiency is corrected. Pica is also seen in mental retardation and psychiatric disturbances such as schizophrenia.

No one is certain why pica occurs, but theories to explain it include an attempt by the body to replace something that's missing (for example, the iron in iron deficiency), a blocking of the sense of smell and taste in conditions of nausea (such as in pregnancy), an infantile hand-to-mouth response to stress or a manifestation of an oral fixation. The tendency to pica runs in families, and the eating of abnormal substances varies considerably from culture to culture, often being incorporated into religious rites, folk medicine and magical beliefs.

Though pica can seem harmless, it often causes significant medical consequences. The substances eaten may produce poisoning within the body (such as phosphorus toxicity from eating match heads, or lead poisoning from eating old paint chips), or may block the absorption of needed nutrients and minerals (the ingestion of clay blocks the normal absorption of iron), or may physically damage the stomach and intestines, leading to abdominal pain and surgery.

Prader-Willi Syndrome

Prader-Willi syndrome (PWS) is an unusual genetic problem due to an abnormality involving the fifteenth chromosome. One of the results is that the area of the brain that normally controls hunger and fullness (the hypothalamus) is not properly developed. Infants with this problem may be unable to feed properly, due to underdeveloped muscles and poor muscle tone. Parents and caregivers have to make continuous efforts to feed them. Then, just prior to school age, these children develop an insatiable appetite. This unstoppable hunger may eventually lead to weight gain so extreme that it causes a life-threatening inability to breathe. The person may be more than 150 percent to 200 percent overweight. This excessive weight gain is also the result of an abnormally low metabolic need for energy. Young adults with PWS will gain weight with a daily intake of only 1,400 calories.

Also seen in this syndrome are signs of mental retardation, short stature and small hands and feet. Behavioral problems, such as temper tantrums as well as verbal and physical aggression, may be present. There may be other peculiarities, such as a high pain threshold, inability to maintain normal body temperature, persistent picking at skin sores and decreased ability to vomit.

Treatment for PWS is lifelong. Refrigerators, cupboards that contain food and even the kitchen itself need to be kept locked. Restricting diets of as low as 600 to 800 calories per day, supplemented by vitamins and calcium, are needed to help reduce the person's weight, to prevent the fatal consequences of this extreme obesity. Individuals may have to be driven from one location to another to prevent them from purchasing food or obtaining it from strangers.

Rumination Disorder

Rumination is the repeated, effortless regurgitation of partially digested food from the stomach back into the mouth. The food is rechewed and swallowed again, or simply spit out.

Unlike repeated vomiting, which may cause heartburn as a result of the high acid content of the vomitus, rumination rarely leads to heartburn. The chewed food is usually brought up very soon after eating, before much stomach acid has been produced. When heartburn does occur, people usually abandon the habit of ruminating.

Rumination may appear in virtually any age group. When it happens in infants as young as three months to one year old, *rumination disorder* may be diagnosed. This abnormal condition may cause weight loss due to malnutrition, and may even lead to death. Rumination disorder may result from neglect or problems with the child-parent relationship. It may also occur in older children who are developmentally delayed (mentally challenged). Except in extreme cases, infants with rumination disorder tend to recover on their own.

Older children, adolescents and adults who *do not* have rumination disorder may sometimes ruminate, especially when depressed or experiencing significant life stress such as family breakup. Rumination also appears in some people with eating disorders; it may begin involuntarily but continue as a learned behavior to control weight. It has been identified in up to 20 percent of those with bulimia, and is probably more common among people with eating disorders than we realize.

Rumination can lead to bad breath (halitosis), erosion of tooth enamel, malnutrition and electrolyte abnormalities. Emotional, family and nutrition counseling, biofeedback and relaxation techniques are among the successful approaches to treatment.

Feeding Disorder of Infancy or Early Childhood

Feeding disorder of infancy or early childhood is demonstrated by a child's persistent inability or refusal to eat adequately, which results in weight loss or an inability to gain weight as expected. This usually occurs before the age of six. The inability to eat is not related to the child's deliberate desire to lose weight due to fear of being obese. Children with this disorder generally recover on their own.

Variant Forms of Anorexia Nervosa and Bulimia Nervosa

Some people severely restrict their food intake and lose large amounts of weight without concern for their weight or for control of their body image. There are no medical reasons for their loss of appetite or weight loss. These individuals have been described by some researchers as having *atypical* anorexia nervosa. Unfortunately, this same term is used by some researchers to describe eating disorders similar to those identified in the "not otherwise specified" classification of eating disorders. For the sake of clarity this form of anorexia nervosa, which is *not* driven by body image, may be called the *variant* form of anorexia nervosa, or simply variant anorexia nervosa.

For example, Emily is a 14-year-old girl who severely restricts what she eats. She eats only hard sugar candies and ice. She is more than 20 percent underweight and has never had her period. She experiences pain in her lower abdomen when she eats or drinks normal foods, and vomits if she feels full after eating only small portions, due to an involuntary urge triggered by nausea. She refuses to eat more because of the sick feeling and abdominal pain she experiences when she eats normally. Emily has always denied deliberately wishing to lose weight, and indeed wishes she could gain weight. Her family and friends have never heard her say that she feels fat, or that she has to go on a diet to lose weight.

Those who have eating disorder behaviors that fit the criteria for bulimia nervosa but have no specific concern for their weight or body image may likewise be described as having *atypical* bulimia nervosa, or the *variant* form of bulimia nervosa (variant bulimia nervosa).

For example, Tina has been binge eating and vomiting for several years. She started to vomit and over-exercise when she was told to lose weight by her ski coach. She had never felt that she was overweight, but she began to lose weight in order to stay on the team. She began bingeing after experiencing severe hunger from vomiting and weight loss. Now that she has left the ski team and has regained her normal weight, she feels comfortable with her body image. She wishes to stop bingeing and vomiting, but she is finding that she cannot stop these behaviors on her own.

FOUR

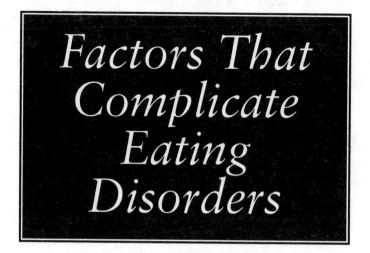

Factors That Complicate Eating Disorders

Jane just can't stop thinking about her weight. She even feels fat in her sleep! She sometimes dreams about binge-ing on food. She is always counting calories. She weighs herself twenty times a day. She looks in the mirror as many times. She is absolutely obsessed with her weight.

Jane is also obsessed with being clean and neat. She compulsively washes her hands until they bleed, and cleans her small apartment six hours a day. She used to wash and clean a great deal before she developed the eating disorder, but these behaviors have become worse since the eating disorder began.

Jane gets so depressed these days that she is unable to keep the nutrition goals she set with her nutritionist. She was doing so well recently, too. She often feels so low that she doesn't want to get out of bed in the morning. She is usually teary and feels that life is hopeless. She used to cut herself with a razor when she was a teenager, but she thought she had escaped that habit. Last night, though, she cut her wrist for the first time in years. She has been using alcohol and smoking marijuana, which helps her to "numb out" and momentarily masks her emotional pain. But the more she uses these drugs, the more depressed she becomes.

Life seemed hard enough a few months ago, with just the eating disorder. Now her escalating depression, obsessive-compulsive tendencies and drug and alcohol use seem out of control. She feels as if she is towing several balls and chains—one for each of her problems. Each problem seems to be getting heavier and heavier, yet no one she knows seems to sense this. Problems that would have been easy to deal with a few months ago are becoming impossible to cope with.

Although some people have an eating disorder as their only important health concern, many have other serious medical, psychological, social or personal problems to deal with. Living with an eating disorder is difficult enough. These other complicating factors can present even further challenges.

Depression

Depression is a mood state that may be expressed by any number of symptoms, such as feelings of worthlessness, sadness, emptiness, irritability, inappropriate guilt, poor sleep, low motivation, weight loss and low sex drive. Feelings of helplessness and hopelessness, poor concentration, excessive sleep, loss of energy and a lack of interest or pleasure can also be present. When a depressed person's loss of appetite persists and results in weight loss, it may be incorrectly attributed to an eating disorder.

Someone who is depressed may have mild, moderate or severe symptoms. The mood state can make people feel anything from a chronic low-grade "blah" to total despair and hopelessness. Depression is the most life-threatening psychological condition associated with an eating disorder, because suicidal thoughts and even suicide attempts are common. Many behavioral changes brought on as a result of depression resemble those associated with eating disorders—social isolation, forgetfulness, irritability, poor decision-making and poor functioning at work or school.

Many people with eating disorders have a family history of mental illness that may include depression, manic depression (bipolar affective disorder) or other emotional problems. Other mental illnesses, such as obsessive-compulsive disorder or schizophrenia, may be present in close relatives.

Although depression may be noticed by others, much of the time it is masked or covered up when the person is in company, which creates the illusion that things are "just fine."

Depression and eating-disorder attitudes and behaviors can show up at different times or at the same time. When a person has both of them together, they can influence each other. Each condition makes it harder to deal with the other one. As an example, when someone is depressed she often feels worse about herself in general, and she may experience heightened self-loathing with regard to body image. Her motivation to recover from the eating disorder wanes and her drive to lose weight becomes dominant. When eating-disorder drives such as urges to binge, purge or lose weight take over, feelings of guilt, shame, being out of control and failure may in turn make the depression worse. Those with a history of depression have a high incidence of alcohol and drug misuse as well.

When someone is dealing with depression and an eating disorder, it is sometimes possible to treat both conditions at the same time. When the depression is too prominent for the eating disorder to be dealt with, the main focus of treatment should be on the depression, since this is the most life-threatening problem.

Depression and eating disorders

"I'm not sure if depression affects my eating disorder or if my eating disorder affects my depression. I think it's a little bit of both. My depression is more or less under control right now due to medication. That's not to say I don't get depressed, because I do. Most of the time I think it's hopeless and I'll never be able to lead a normal life. I've already spent half my life with an eating disorder, and that thought in itself is depressing."

Seasonal Affective Disorder

Seasonal affective disorder (SAD) is a state of cyclic depression that seems to develop as a result of the changes of season. It is felt that the reduced sunlight available in autumn and winter changes the mood and emotions of some people drastically, producing feelings of depression. SAD typically increases as fall turns into winter, and it is no coincidence that eating-disorder behaviors may reappear or get worse during these times. SAD often aggravates poor body-image feelings, and the eating disorder becomes a familiar way of coping with these feelings as well as with depression. During periods of SAD, self-harm and suicide attempts become more prevalent. The best treatment is regular exposure to sunlight. Long walks outdoors, even during gray winter days, may provide relief. SAD can be treated with exposure to specially constructed artificial lights that mimic the illumination from the sun. Antidepressants are also used.

Obsessive-Compulsive Disorder

Obsessions are recurrent and intrusive thoughts, feelings, ideas or sensations. They constantly fill the mind despite any effort you make to dislodge them. Compulsions are conscious, recurrent, irresistible urges to perform certain acts. Since compulsions are the actions resulting from obsessions, obsessions increase a person's anxiety, while compulsions reduce the anxiety.

Obsessions and compulsions are common traits that many people experience. When they do not especially influence someone's life, they are referred to as obsessive traits and compulsive traits. When they are more persistent and affect someone's life significantly, they are considered an obsessive-compulsive disorder.

Common obsessive thoughts are such things as over-concern with self-doubts or contamination. Common compulsions include excessive washing of the body, counting, cleaning the home, inappropriate frequent flicking of light switches, and repeatedly checking that doors are locked or that a stove has been turned off.

Obsessive-compulsive traits and disorders are common in those with eating disorders, and are often associated with poor body image and weight and food control. These people are obsessed with being "too fat," wanting to lose weight, and fearing overeating, and they feel a compulsion to over-exercise, restrict their food intake or use laxatives. Some say they are obsessed about body image, weight and food for over 90 percent of the day, and their compulsions may lead to exercising many hours a day, weighing or looking in a mirror ten times a day, bingeing and vomiting dozens of times or not eating for days. Obsessive-compulsive-like traits often cause people with eating disorders to brood about their body image, weight and food control at times when they want to forget about them, and sometimes make them do things even though they desperately want not to. These obsessive-compulsive traits, which may be very powerful, do not represent a true obsessive-compulsive disorder, but people who have the tendencies are often misdiagnosed as having such a disorder, and the misdiagnosis can complicate treatment of the eating disorder.

Personality Disorders

Personality is the combination of emotional and behavioral traits that characterize a person. These traits are normally stable and predictable, but people with personality disorders exhibit emotional and behavioral traits that are often abnormal and inflexible, and prevent them from being happy and successful, from adjusting to society.

One type of personality disorder that may be present in someone with an eating disorder is borderline personality disorder. A person with this disorder may show a persistent pattern of impulsiveness and instability in interpersonal relationships, as well as poor self-image and rapidly changing mood. Such a pattern is usually evident by early adulthood. Many people with the disorder try to avoid imagined or perceived abandonment. Their relationships with others may be intense, but are often abnormal—relationships may be overvalued (idealized) or undervalued: other people are seen as all good or all bad. Relationships are often unstable, and there is a history of failed friendships and partnerships. Impulsive spending, multiple sexual encounters or drug use may be seen. Some of these people feel chronic emptiness or loneliness, intense anger, anxiety, irritability or sadness. Persistent self-loathing and suicidal thoughts followed by suicide attempts and self-mutilation (cutting, hitting or burning) are common. Paranoia (feelings of being persecuted or scrutinized) and dissociative symptoms (feelings of being outside one's body, or even being a completely separate person) are possible. Note, however, that many of these feelings and behaviors are common to adolescents, and therefore a diagnosis of borderline personality disorder should not be made for someone in this age group.

The borderline personality disorder (BPD) may itself prevent people from accepting help from others, due to a fear of being disappointed or abandoned by friends and caregivers. Sometimes there is a feeling of not being worthy of help, or a fear of further failure. Depressive symptoms or a focus on self-harm prevents some people from moving forward with recovery. Impulsive behaviors such as switching therapists frequently, skipping a job interview or stopping medication may interrupt established plans that would otherwise help. Someone who is constantly confronting one life crisis (a new job, new home or new relationship) after another will find it difficult to focus on more long-term improvement. Because some of the behaviors of people with BPD are similar to behaviors caused by other conditions, the disorder can be confused with major depression, bipolar disorder or schizophrenia, as well as with other personality disorders. Careful evaluation by experienced physicians is needed, as making the wrong diagnosis—or simply failing to make the right one—leads to confusion and inappropriate treatment.

Although a borderline personality disorder may present many obstacles, it need not prevent someone from recovering from an eating disorder, nor does it mean that borderline attitudes and behaviors cannot be improved with appropriate support from professionals, friends and family. It is encouraging to see how borderline traits lessen or disappear with support and treatment.

Bipolar Disorders

Bipolar disorders—more commonly known as manic-depressive disorders—are so called because people suffering from them have two extremes, or poles, of mood: depression and mania. Mania is a state in which a person may feel unusually and unrealistically positive about herself and life in general. Her sense of self-esteem is inflated and grandiose. Usually, she is filled with energy and needs little sleep. She may spend recklessly, be sexually promiscuous or otherwise behave inappropriately, which could lead to painful consequences. Her ideas may fly or race. Delusions or hallucinations may be present. This behavior alternates with the other extreme, depression.

When someone with an eating disorder has a bipolar disorder as well, the bipolar conditions may interfere with progress in treating the eating disorder, because the person may experience profound depressive symptoms that resist typical antidepressants. If the diagnosis is not properly made, inappropriate treatments—usually inappropriate counseling and medication—may be tried.

Schizophrenia

Schizophrenia is a mental disorder marked by a breakdown in the relationship between thoughts, feelings and actions. The cause of schizophrenia is unknown, but it can produce symptoms of confusion, disorientation, delusions, hallucination and paranoia, and disorganized and incoherent speech. When someone with an eating disorder also happens to have schizophrenia, it certainly complicates the problem. Until an accurate diagnosis has been made, someone with schizophrenia may be mistakenly diagnosed as having a major depressive illness, bipolar disorder or borderline personality disorder, since all of these other conditions can mimic the behavior seen in schizophrenia. Although there is no cure for schizophrenia, there are medications that can significantly improve functioning. When schizophrenia symptoms are under control, treatment and support for an eating disorder can be considered.

Drug Abuse

Prescription drugs, over-the-counter drugs and "street drugs" can all be misused by people with eating disorders. Some drugs are used for their ability to get someone "stoned" or high, or as stimulants or "uppers." Other drugs are used to help people deal with their body-image-control problems by suppressing their appetite or making them too "stoned" to eat. Some drugs are used for both purposes.

Drugs such as cocaine, heroin and amphetamines are sometimes used to control weight, and may therefore be used by those with eating disorders. All have dangers attached. Some are injected through hypodermic needles; if needles are shared, they can transmit hepatitis, which increases the chance of liver failure due to cirrhosis of the liver, and liver cancer. Sharing needles can also spread HIV, leading to AIDS. People with these diseases may be unable to get disability or life insurance, which can lead to catastrophic financial costs. Marijuana can temporarily preoccupy someone trying to avoid eating, but it will likely stimulate hunger and lead to hearty eating. Hallucinogenic drugs such as LSD, mescaline and MDA may delay eating by preoccupying the person or temporarily suppressing hunger, but after the trip back to earth, the food will still be waiting.

Prescription drugs may be acquired legally from a physician or purchased illegally. Many prescription drugs that have a street value are chemically addicting. Most prescription drugs abused in this way are purchased by someone who plans to get "stoned" or sedated, but some have the potential to cause temporary weight loss by suppressing the appetite. Many of these drugs, known as stimulants, are related to amphetamines, or "speed," and have marked effects (racing thoughts, rapid heartbeat, emotional instability) other than appetite suppression. Appetite suppressants either do not work at all or have very short-lived success in controlling weight.

Almost all these drugs can be dangerous, especially when used by someone with the serious emotional or medical complications of eating disorders. Many of these drugs profoundly worsen depression and increase the risk of suicide. Some can lead to life-threatening problems with the rhythm and contracting ability of the heart.

Alcohol Abuse

Alcohol is a drug, but one that is largely socially acceptable and legal for those of age. Like food, it is often an integral part of social and family functions. Alcohol abuse is common among people with eating disorders. Alcohol may be used to temporarily suppress appetite, and to cause intoxication, to fend off thoughts of food. Alcohol may also be used to induce longer sleeping periods, which leave fewer hours a day available to focus on food. However, alcohol itself contains a lot of calories.

Alcohol is addicting. It worsens depression and increases the risk of suicide. As long as people are actively drinking, treatment for an eating disorder alone is pointless. Alcohol and drug-dependence problems must generally be treated before eating-disorder problems, because of their chaotic influence on appetite, reasoning ability and emotions.

Pregnancy

Most women strive to have the healthiest pregnancy and labor possible, through a combination of healthy eating, exercise, vitamin and mineral supplements and the avoidance of harmful drugs and alcohol. When the woman has an eating disorder, however, behaviors such as dieting to lose weight, vomiting, bingeing and laxative abuse can put both the mother and the fetus at great risk. Weight loss, or the lack of weight gain expected during pregnancy, can result in an undernourished fetus, putting the baby at risk of medical problems.

Vomiting, and use of laxatives and diuretics, may produce serious electrolyte abnormalities that could lead to the woman falling or fainting, or could even cause sudden death because the function of the heart has been disturbed. The fetus itself may not receive adequate nutrition. A pregnant woman whose weight gain is not adequate, or whose eating-disorder behaviors (such as vomiting) are significantly out of control, may have to be admitted to hospital. Meal support and intravenous fluids to correct electrolyte abnormalities can be most helpful.

Diabetes

Diabetes is a medical condition that results in the body not being able to metabolize sugar (glucose) properly. Insulin, a hormone naturally produced by the human pancreas, is essential to the body's proper use of sugar. The diabetic may not produce sufficient insulin or may produce none at all, or the insulin may not be effective due to insulin resistance, depending on which type of diabetes she has.

Without the help of insulin, the glucose in the blood is not able to enter the cells of various organs. As a result, the level of glucose in the blood becomes excessively high. This high-glucose state, called hyperglycemia, results in weakness, dizziness, falling or even coma. Some organs, such as the kidneys

---

About diabetes

Type 1 diabetes, which is most often identified in young adults, adolescents and children, requires not only healthy nutrition and exercise management but also insulin injections. The amount of insulin must be carefully balanced against the amount of food (supplying sugar) and the amount of exercise (burning sugar off as energy).

Type 2 diabetes, usually seen in older adults, can initially be treated with adequate nutrition and exercise programs. Often, pills that help the body metabolize glucose properly are used. Sometimes, insulin injections are used as well.

and eyes, can become irreversibly damaged if proper diabetic control is not maintained.

Diabetes and an eating disorder make a particularly difficult and dangerous combination. Since diabetics typically require fairly strict nutrition control—that is, they need consistently sized meals with very little sugar content—restricting, bingeing and purging make good diabetic control impossible. For example, someone restricting her food requires less insulin than she needs during healthy eating periods. Someone on a binge will consume far too many calories for the insulin dose that normally controls her blood glucose. Vomiting removes an unpredictable amount of nutrition, so that it's impossible to calculate the right insulin dose. Over-exercising or under-exercising can also disproportionately lower or raise blood glucose levels. A low blood glucose level will produce a feeling of hunger; a high blood glucose level will decrease appetite.

If a diabetic does not monitor her blood glucose levels several times a day while she is subject to eating disorder behaviors, she will not know how much insulin or other diabetes medication to use. Some people even skip their insulin, because they know this will lead to a very high blood glucose level, which will cause the body to void large concentrations of glucose in urine; the loss of water will create a temporary weight loss, and the loss of glucose is seen as a diet technique. Skipping insulin is a *very dangerous eating-disorder behavior* and should be treated as a medical emergency. An imbalance between insulin and glucose—too much insulin *or* too little insulin—can lead to death.

Sexual Abuse
Sexual abuse may be a complicating factor in eating disorders. It can happen to either females or males, and the perpetrator

can be of either sex. Sexual abuse may happen at any age from infancy into adulthood, and can precede the development of the eating disorder or take place after it begins.

Someone who has been sexually abused shares many of the feelings of someone with an eating disorder—shame, guilt, depression and a sense of not having control over life. Sexual abuse, specifically, causes someone to feel shame and guilt over having been assaulted. The abused person may have low self-esteem and a feeling of not being worthy. She may feel that, in some way, she was at least partially to blame for the abuse, and that she therefore cannot share her experience with others.

Body image is most certainly affected, as the body has become the focus of markedly decreased self-worth. Sexual abuse makes the body an object of power, because someone else now has power over the body and its emotions. It reduces the perceived value of the person to that of the physical being, undermining the importance of feelings.

Some people who have been sexually abused have problems surface later in life, when nightmares, flashbacks and overpowering feelings of depression and panic, or revulsion at physical intimacy, appear. Post-traumatic stress disorder can result, and a profound inability to cope. Some people are unable to work, study or take care of their children. Body-image-control feelings and behaviors related to eating disorders can become much worse, or may actually improve temporarily during post-traumatic stress disorder. Those who have experienced sexual abuse are at increased risk of alcohol and drug addictions.

If sexual abuse is an issue, it must be dealt with. It cannot remain a secret and be left unattended. If you have a history of sexual abuse, you need to have your experiences and feelings validated by talking to someone who believes you and assures you that what you feel is truly important and worthy of attention. You need to know that it was not your fault. Trauma related to sexual abuse may often be treated while you receive treatment for your eating disorder. Sometimes, however, the abuse issues must receive treatment first, so that you will have the time and energy to focus upon your eating-disorder concerns at a later date.

FIVE

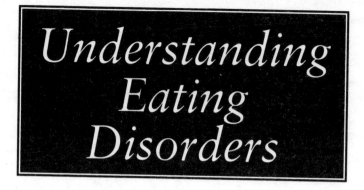

Understanding Eating Disorders

Robert loved to run. He had always wanted to compete in a marathon, and had trained for years to this end. One day he seriously twisted his ankle. The injury was so bad that he was unable to train for months. He became depressed and despondent over the prospect of never being able to run competitively again. He started to gain weight due to being less active. Friends teased him about his "beer gut." Having always prided himself on being fit, he now began to feel he was letting himself go. He developed a desperate need to keep his weight down, and started to diet. He became a vegetarian and began to skip meals. He started to work out more and more often, using exercises that did not put much strain on his sore ankle. He went to the gym daily and used the stationary bike, rowing machine and weights. He did countless sit-ups and push-ups.

Robert lost weight month after month, until he looked like a skeleton. His skin was sallow—a sickening yellow color. Friends became very worried and his boss even asked him if he needed to take some sick leave. Robert declined; he felt

91

that he was performing well and saw no need for concern. He became more isolated. He would not go out with friends or return their phone calls because he knew they would comment about his weight. He even lost interest in his girlfriend. He had no sex drive anymore, and found it too much of an effort to keep the peace between them. Besides, she was always nagging him about his eating and his exercise.

Robert also avoided his family as much as he could. His father had always denigrated him and Robert had never felt that he could please him. Even getting a law degree wasn't enough—his father hadn't shown up for his graduation. His mother had always smothered him and tried to protect him from the world. These days, he just wanted everyone in his life to leave him alone.

One day, Robert woke up in a hospital emergency room. He had fainted at work and hit his head on the ground. His chin was cut and his tongue required several stitches. The doctor told him that he had developed a near-fatal heart rhythm and was lucky to be alive. The doctor blamed Robert's brush with death on anorexia nervosa. He told Robert that his liver enzymes were critically elevated and asked him if he knew why. Robert admitted that he had been injecting himself with anabolic steroids—a habit he'd picked up from other athletes. The doctor explained the health risks of steroid use—infertility, irreversible liver damage, liver cancer.

When Robert felt a bit better, he left the emergency room. He went home, cleaned himself up and drove directly to the gym.

Many people seek to understand why they developed an eating disorder. They realize that people in our society often place an abnormal value on weight and appearance, and that many people diet. They wonder why *they* developed this complicated, abnormal pattern of behavior while others did not. The answer to this question is usually not a simple one, because eating disorders are complicated and very individual. Usually they occur as a result of many factors and forces. However, understanding the pattern of these forces and influences, and their dynamics, allows us to begin to make sense of the problem.

In the development of an eating disorder, internal factors such as genetics, biochemical makeup and personality traits combine with external pressure from family, peers and society. Although one or more of these influences may be more prominent in one person than in another, it is usually the combination that leads to the disorder, rather than one single event or personality trait. Some people are predisposed (because of their genetics and personality) to developing an eating disorder. Others, by their makeup, are much more resistant.

The Influence of the Media

The media—particularly television, magazines and movies—are an important force in our culture, and are felt to be part of the reason some people develop eating disorders. We are constantly bombarded by images of thinness, vitality and youth that, for many people, are irresistible, though completely unattainable and unrealistic. This bombardment produces a feeling of dissatisfaction with ourselves and our bodies, and this dissatisfaction is quickly and fervently addressed by the same media—they show us endless ways we can improve ourselves. Advertisements seem to say, "You could be better than you are if you just changed this or that about yourself." "After all," the message reads, "you're no good as you are. You're too fat, too short, not physically attractive enough, too old. You should change, and then you'll be truly happy!" The artificial image of what we should look like, and the ways we can attain that image, are foisted upon us ad nauseam, despite the fact that the image is an abnormal one.

In many places—such as Africa, where advertising is not nearly as prominent or powerful—the ideal image is completely different. In West Africa, for example, the ideal female image has a healthy proportion of subcutaneous fat, with larger buttocks and fuller breasts. This image is realistic and healthy.

The "ideal" female in the Western media version is exceptionally tall and abnormally thin, which is a state very few women can achieve. In one study, the ideal photographer's model was found to be 5'10" (178 cm) tall and to weigh 110 pounds (50 kg). This is ridiculously abnormal. The same distorted image applies to men. The media's "ideal" body image for them is tall and trim, with prominent muscles and a very low percentage of body fat.

It's a seductive process; thinness and beauty promise many things. You will be respected, more successful, sexier, we are told. You will look more confident, be more self-assured, have

The Barbie-doll syndrome

For many girls in our society, playing with dolls is an enjoyable and seemingly innocent part of childhood. The Barbie doll is one of the most successful toys ever conceived; eight hundred million Barbie dolls have been sold worldwide and annual sales top one billion dollars. The doll allows endless hours of pleasure for girls who dress and undress it, groom and beautify it, and then admire it.

However, the Barbie doll (and Ken, the male counterpart) are highly unrealistic models for shape and weight. For an average female of 5'2" and 125 pounds (157 cm and 57 kg) to attain the "look" of Barbie, she would have to grow 24 inches (61 cm) in height, expand 5 inches (13 cm) in her chest circumference and decrease 6 inches (15 cm) in her waist. For an average male 6 feet tall and 185 pounds (183 cm and 84 kg) to attain the "look" of Ken, he would have to grow 20 inches (51 cm) in height and add 10 inches (25 cm) to his waist and 8 inches (20 cm) in his chest. Obviously there is a large discrepancy between the body proportions for healthy, normal subjects and these ubiquitous dolls. If the dolls are used as standards for comparison, discontent or even despair may be the result.

more self-esteem. The ideal supposedly confers power, youth-fulness and a sense of being in control. You are promised the envy of those unable to achieve the ideal.

Pick up any fashion magazine, look at the publicity photos for theatrical or musical events, or look closely at television and movie stars. Images of thinness, vitality and perfect align-ment with the advertising ideal are everywhere. These people look abnormal, and often they have even had plastic surgery to maintain this abnormal ideal. Sometimes the images are obvious and overpowering, but more often, day in and day out, they are pervasive and subliminal, establishing them-selves in our subconscious minds in a nebulous but danger-ous association with happiness and success.

In a similar manner, we are bombarded by advertisements for food that influence our attitude to eating and weight. At dinnertime, television advertises relatively cheap, high-calorie, appealing food already prepared and waiting for you a short car ride or bike ride away, at any number of fast-food restau-rants. Many food ads in magazines and tabloids now include promises of "low-fat" or "low-cholesterol" ways to satisfy hunger; that is, you can apparently eat without putting on weight. Paradoxically, interspersed among the food ads are weight-loss ads, often featuring actors who do not appear ever to have needed to lose weight! The juxtaposition of these ads parallels the cycling of bingeing and purging seen in bulimia.

Catering to our desire to achieve weight loss and to match the media's ideal, fad diets are ever-present and always chang-ing. Many fad diets are dangerously unbalanced, such as those with high protein or high carbohydrate ratios, or water diets, grapefruit diets or cider vinegar diets. They typically leave out significant portions of important food groups, and they rarely allow sufficient daily energy intake to prevent hunger. Although you can lose weight for a short time on fad diets,

The set-point theory of weight

Evidence is emerging that the human body is programmed to be a specific weight at given ages. The set-point theory of weight states that, like our height, eye color and intelligence, our weight is genetically determined. Although we can increase or decrease it to some degree, it will always tend to return to its predetermined level. This is one of the reasons weight-loss diets have a failure rate over 95 percent, in the long term.

Our weight characteristics are often similar to those of our parents. The genes that determine weight come from several chromosomes. The "set point" can be affected by early childhood eating habits, physical activity, illness and drugs. By and large, however, the set point determines our weight.

If you speak to overweight people who have been on several diets over the years, most will tell you that they wish they had never started dieting in the first place. After every diet in which they lose weight, they gain it back, and often they gain weight above the point where they were when they started the diet. They try harder to diet the next time, but experience the same yo-yo pattern of weight loss and rebound weight gain. As someone said, "I'd be half the person I am today if only I hadn't dieted."

Often, people say that when they started to diet they had to restrict their food only a little bit, or exercise a little bit, to lose weight. After many diets, much more starving and exercising may not result in them losing even a little weight. This is because, when the body has starved, it tries to defend itself against starvation in the future by improving its ability to store fat. In other words, dieting teaches the body to store fat in fat cells more easily and more quickly. The bottom line is that dieting leads to obesity. Diets do not work!

they produce such hunger that, when the diet is over, the body often overeats as compensation. The cycling of diet and overeating continues and ultimately has the opposite effect: over several years you gain weight.

The media have also "discovered" eating disorders, and glorified them. Talk-show hosts present guests with eating disorders, to create a sensation at the expense of these people and their families. The presentation of an emaciated girl with anorexia nervosa, hanging onto life by a thread, creates a powerful image, and the tears of the audience flow—and

Miss (Anorexic) America

Beauty contests offer us an objective assessment of what our society sees as desirable physical qualities in females. A clear shift toward a thinner "ideal" shape for women in Western culture is evident from statistics for the Miss America Pageant over the last several years.

Researchers used the height and weight of contestants to calculate their body mass index (BMI), and learned that contestants' BMI has fallen over the years. (See the BMI chart in Chapter 1, "Anorexia Nervosa.") In the 1920s contestants had BMIs in the normal range, but since the 1950s the BMI of contestants has been falling steadily. From 1970 to 1978, on average, these beauty contestants were 15 percent lighter than the average weight for the rest of the females in the country.

What this analysis shows is that our ideal of beauty in women has changed dramatically. We are idealizing and rewarding a thinness that is unhealthy and unachievable for most women.

ratings rise. But instead of educating the public about the negative aspects of eating disorders, this image has the opposite effect: it teaches onlookers how to lose weight dramatically. Vulnerable young people do not see the horrors that anorexia nervosa and bulimia can bring. Instead, they are impressed that someone can eat "all she wants" and yet lose weight just by sticking a finger down her throat and vomiting. Only the most extreme, most graphic forms of eating-disorder behaviors and body wasting are presented on television, not the much more common and milder forms. Moreover, these cases are usually presented in a pathetic light, implying that the conditions are completely hopeless and there is no chance of recovery. The presentation rarely makes the point that these are complicated yet *reversible* conditions. The eating disorders are exploited for their visual and emotional impact on the audience, not in any attempt to create understanding of the problem, or sympathy for it. Such programs are glorified "freak shows" designed and broadcast for their shock value alone.

Exercise Trends

The last couple of decades have brought a major increase in personal exercise in our society, with more of us taking up sporting activities—both on teams and as individuals. This is laudable because some physical activity is essential to health and well-being. On television we see world-class athletes close up, in their sports and in their personal lives. They are made to seem "just like us" and they make us think, "I could do that if I would only work harder at it." The competitive basis of sports is emphasized, and extremes of exercise endurance are made attractive. Instead of exercising at our own reasonable level for the sake of physical activity, we are led to see exercise as a route to glamor and success.

Exercise has also been glorified as a method of weight loss and weight control, and many eating-disorder patients abuse it. In fact, exercise itself can become a serious eating-disorder behavior. People with exercise compulsions can be even more resistant to treatment than those with anorexia and bulimia.

The significance of weight in some sports is an important factor in the development of eating disorders. Some of the pressure to lose weight is due to strict weight guidelines set by athletic coaches and organizations. Whole teams have reported having dieting and bulimic behaviors imposed on them so that they would meet weight goals necessary to be allowed to remain on the team. The higher the level of competition, the more intense the pressure to maintain or lower weight, in spite of the increasing muscle bulk that is a result of the training. For example, the categories of competitive rowing are based on weight. To be in the lightweight category a rower must be less than 125 pounds (about 57 kg); a rower over this weight must compete in the heavyweight category. There is no medium-weight category, and the heavyweight category is usually filled by larger, stronger athletes.

Consequently, rowers sometimes adopt eating-disorder behaviors just to be able to enter the light category, where they perceive their chances of winning to be better. Wrestlers and boxers face the same kind of pressure.

In other sports, such as competitive swimming, there are no defined weight categories, but coaches pressure athletes because they believe that the best performance comes from a lean athlete with a lower percentage of body fat. Daily weigh-ins in front of other team members create embarrassment and fear, and focus the athletes' attention on body image and eating habits. Expulsion from a swim team, whether it be high school, university or world class, could have a serious impact on the swimmer's self-worth, identity and even career. Therefore, swimmers starve themselves, vomit, or use laxatives or other mechanisms to maintain their weight at the lowest level possible.

Sometimes the pressure is less obvious. In sports where weight categories are not a requirement, there is still pressure to look good on television or to gain a competitive edge over the other players. Someone who plays a team sport such as curling or hockey may be expected to maintain a lower weight just for the sake of psychological advantage.

In addition, serious athletes who develop sports-related injuries often try to compensate for not being able to exercise as much as they used to. The fear of weight gain is significant for them, because their inability to train regularly may decrease their muscle mass and increase the amount of fat in their bodies. They may try to compensate for this by eating abnormally. For example, runners who sprain their ankles or develop overuse injuries in their knees or backs may transfer their energies to weightlifting and stationary bicycle work, but may find that they still have to diet severely, or purge with vomiting or laxatives, just to keep their weight down.

Genetic Predisposition

Anorexia nervosa and bulimia nervosa run in families, and genetic factors may play a significant role. From studies with twins it appears that specific genetic factors are more important in anorexia nervosa than in bulimia; in the latter there seems to be a more general predisposition to the cycle of overeating and purging. Many studies report an increased rate of eating disorders among first-degree relatives (parent, child, sibling) of those with anorexia nervosa or bulimia. Similarly, female relatives of a person with anorexia nervosa have a tenfold greater risk of developing an eating disorder than the general population, and even second-degree relatives have an increased risk. However, though the genetic predisposition may be present, it will not produce an eating disorder by itself, but only in combination with the other factors listed in this chapter.

Specific Personality Traits

Each of us has a distinct combination of qualities and characteristics that makes us different. This is our personality, our identity, and it includes our attitudes, experiences and outlook. Although the personalities of those with eating disorders can span the entire spectrum of human characteristics, some traits are more commonly seen.

Low Self-Esteem

Quite consistently, low self-esteem emerges as a powerful (sometimes overwhelming) perception among those with eating disorders. An adequate sense of self-worth is a very important acquisition as a child ages and matures. Failure to develop this often produces feelings of worthlessness, unhappiness and dissatisfaction. The presence of a well-developed sense of personal worth or value allows you to function well throughout life. It acts as a reserve or support in times of

Living with an eating disorder

"My eating disorder obliterates the real me."

"It ridicules me. I've played the game over and over again, the one where I have a cookie from the cupboard, or a candy or a drink of a tasty juice (whatever the item) and tell myself, 'I'll only have one or two.' Then I close the container ... only to find myself returning for more."

"It restricts my social life. I don't like to go to parties or banquets where I'll be expected to eat. I check where the bathroom is so I can purge. I'm relieved if it's a single bathroom so I can have privacy."

"It wrecks my teeth. I spend a lot of time in the dentist's chair."

"I have osteoporosis in my back and hips. I have pain most of the time."

stress, disappointment or vulnerability. Lacking this, many people with eating disorders turn in on themselves, questioning their own value. Some researchers and psychologists believe that this lack of self-esteem lies at the heart of eating disorders. Someone may be an excellent student, an athlete or very likable, but if the individual sees himself or herself as unaccomplished, socially unacceptable or a failure, there is no pleasure derived from interactions with others, or from accomplishments. Accolades from teachers, family and friends do little to diminish the self-reproach. Although others may think she "has it all," a girl without self-esteem may feel she has nothing of value to offer the world. She is blind to her own strengths and abilities, even though others can easily see them. A good sense of your own distinctive qualities, the things you are good at, and your own worth gives you the personal strength and momentum to carry on through the stresses and strains of life.

Perfectionism

A perfectionist is a person who will accept nothing less than the absolutely faultless completion of a task. Perfectionists have developed a rigid sense of what is acceptable, and they are much more exacting and demanding than others. They are very strict with themselves, and have practiced the discipline of self-denial, so they are able to achieve their "perfect" solution to many of life's problems and challenges. They find themselves upset and unhappy when one of their arbitrarily perfect goals is not reached. Often, personal accomplishments of a very high standard are seen as not good enough. The A received in an English exam can bring great disappointment and self-recrimination to someone who expected an A+. Perfectionists are often self-effacing, and devalue their high marks or other accomplishments by comments such as "That was just an easy exam," or "I don't really deserve that mark." Their standards are set so high that failure is inevitable. They spend their lives as failures, only rarely able to achieve the perfection that their personality demands. Sometimes perfectionism leads to procrastination as the fear of failure builds.

Perfectionists demand the same high standards of others as of themselves. When parents, teachers, friends and partners can't meet their high expectations, they come to feel perpetual disappointment in these others. Nothing is ever good enough to satisfy their inappropriate drive.

Unfortunately, failure is a very painful experience for perfectionists. This combination of setting an unattainably high standard and being very sensitive to the unavoidable failure is an important factor in eating disorders, as it often fuels the person's poor sense of worth and low self-esteem. Although perfectionists strive for perfection, they see themselves as imperfect, and their continual attempts to reach perfection are a daily source of anxiety, disappointment and unhappiness. They lack the ability to see a wider picture, to realize that many times their goals are not appropriate, and are, in fact, self-destructive.

Perfectionism and eating disorders

"I am definitely a perfectionist. This creates very high standards for my body weight and performance level. If either of those was less than perfect, I would deal with the resulting low self-esteem and disappointment by bingeing. This would create increased disgust in myself and I would sink into a deep hole. The only way out of the hole is to once again be 'perfect'—setting myself up for the inevitable fall once again."

"I don't think I'm a real perfectionist but I certainly try to make some things perfect. I guess the beginning of my anorexia was my striving for a perfect body. It didn't work. Most things that I try to be perfect about don't work."

Emotional Sensitivity

Many people who suffer from eating disorders are very sensitive to the needs and feelings of others, and are responsive to them. It is a helpful and laudable personality trait, but too often those who are extremely sensitive want to help others at the expense of their own needs. They notice the emotional pain in others, yet do not recognize their own. They feel that others come first and they may not allow their own emotional needs to be met (or even acknowledged). This type of person places great value on "keeping the peace," and on placating and satisfying others' emotional needs while denying her own. These are often "perfect children," the ones who don't cause any difficulty, have no emotional outbursts, make no demands that their personal needs be met; the ones who are easily managed, without confrontation or crisis, throughout their childhood. As young people they are often the easiest ones to parent, because they rarely challenge the decisions and directions given to them. They perceive that the meeting of their own needs is very much secondary to the meeting of the needs of their family and parents, and they rarely insist on a personal stance or priority. It's hard to get them to state their feelings (especially negative feelings), because they feel that this would make others around them unhappy, and they derive quite a bit of pleasure in life from making others happy, often to the extent that they themselves are unhappy. They tend to feel that their emotional needs are somehow not as deserving as those of others in the immediate family. They have difficulty insisting that their own needs, desires and hopes be addressed and validated.

What Function Does the Eating Disorder Serve?

When someone has the genetic tendency and the personality traits discussed above, the stage is set for the development of an eating disorder. However, only a small percentage of people with this combination of predisposing factors actually develop an eating disorder. What makes this happen in some people and not in others?

Research has determined that there is something about the process of losing weight that offers some of these young people something that is desirable, something that has eluded them before, something that gives them positive reinforcement. Somehow the realization that they are able to lose weight makes them feel better about themselves, and this pleasant, positive feeling is what makes the behavior continue. They have developed a personal gain because of their weight loss. It is worth looking at this aspect of personal gain in some detail, because it is inherently associated with perpetuation of the behavior.

Eating Disorders Give Some People Control

If you had to choose a single word to explain eating disorders, that word would be "control." People who develop eating disorders have a desperate need for control that they have not previously found in their lives. They see themselves as passive, powerless, their lives controlled by others and by events beyond their influence. This feeling of helplessness is very upsetting. It makes them intensely unhappy, and they seek some method of regaining control and direction.

Initially, the person wishes to control her food intake, perhaps because she perceives herself to be overweight, or because she has accepted the media's message that she would be happier with a different body image. Like many of us, she begins to diet, but something soon happens that makes the dieting irreversible. She finds that she is good at dieting, that—probably because of her tendency to be a perfectionist, and her ability to deny her own needs and wants—the weight loss is relatively easy to achieve. The diet has thus functioned as a mechanism to "control" weight. She may feel that this is the only aspect of life she has been able to so easily control. Having direction over at least a minor part of life feels like an accomplishment, and she is happy about it. She (or he—remember that 5 to 10 percent of those with eating disorders are male) continues to diet.

Soon friends and family notice the weight loss and, at least at first, they praise the dieter, impressed with her "control" over her "weight problem" and envious that she has been able to achieve such a weight loss. After all, they know how difficult it is to lose weight and keep it off. This praise reinforces the idea in the dieter's mind that she has developed control over this aspect of life. As the dieting continues, reinforced by the feelings of success, the sense of control can be extended from herself to others around her. Very little will bring her the same attention from her parents as the marked weight loss that eventually becomes evident. Likewise, the smell of vomit in the washroom will lead to a confrontation with parents after the dieter has assured them that the eating disorder has disappeared. In a bizarre way, the dieter has manipulated the situation—"controlled it"—

to make her family and friends express their concern and love for her.

A sense of control also extends to feelings such as anger, fear, anxiety, shame or guilt. During bingeing episodes, many bulimics say that they "numb out," meaning that they enter a state that temporarily removes them (or at least protects them) from negative emotions and feelings. They give in to their overwhelming desire to eat, but they spare themselves the self-recrimination and unhappiness that this activity would normally produce. They describe the bulimic episode as a blur, and the next day they have a difficult time remembering what they ate or how many times they vomited.

Similarly, the eating disorder "controls" their deeper feelings of being unworthy. Many people with eating disorders say they hear voices in their heads that tell them they are bad or a failure or otherwise unacceptable. Unless they continue the eating disorder, the harshness and frequency of the negative voices, and the turmoil they bring, only become worse. Sometimes, as people are trying to give up their eating disorders, this internal dialogue can be so intense as to be intolerable. Many times, they objectify this negative force as "something inside me" or "a very powerful voice" or some other depersonalized description. They perceive it as being not a part of themselves but something foreign, something demanding and directing. Only by perpetuating the eating disorder can they "control" these self-destructive and self-punishing psychological forces.

Excuses such as "She's sick, she can't go out to dinner with us" allow the dieter control over encounters that might be emotionally painful. Having an eating disorder allows you to be excused from many of life's expectations, such as attending classes, studying, seeking employment, dating, forming relationships and other socializing. It thus becomes a way of

What makes eating disorders worse?

"I went to an eating-disorders workshop that was purely informational. I was very well read in the area and I had all the right answers. However, the workshop didn't help at all. The problem was, it kept the disorder at an intellectual level—a place I was quite familiar with. It was my body and especially my feelings that I needed to get in touch with—this is what has made the difference for me."

"It makes it worse if I step on the scale in the morning and find myself up a pound or two. Depression makes it worse, but it can go either way with me. It can increase my binges and purges or it can make me eat less."

"The eating disorder gets worse when I hate myself more. I hate myself when I'm engaged in activities that are meaningless to me."

avoiding failure. It "controls" your life because it prevents you (by giving you a "medical reason") from being exposed to situations where your feelings of inferiority and helplessness might be reinforced. This is particularly significant for a person with perfectionist tendencies and a poor sense of self-worth. If you can't do something because of an illness, you can't feel guilty about not being able to achieve perfection.

Identity As a Perpetuating Factor

With the passage of time an individual's very identity may become incorporated into the eating disorder. The eating disorder is all-pervasive and all-consuming, and the person no longer maintains his or her own identity, but takes on the identity of the disorder, becoming "someone with anorexia nervosa." The sufferer thinks constantly about food, body image and control. Other aspects of life (such as social contact, friends and family, work and school) become less important and sometimes the person feels, "What am I without my eating disorder? Who am I without it? Everyone knows me as Mary the bulimic!" As the pattern continues for months or years, the idea of giving up the eating disorder becomes extremely threaten-ing because the anorexic or bulimic cannot imagine life without it—cannot conceive of her identity without it. She may feel that others will not be able to relate to her if she recovers.

We all have our own sense of identity. It's often associated with where we are in school, what sort of work we do, and external measurements of how we fit into society, rather than internal personal qualities. In this case the identity of being an athlete, a good student, an accomplished musician or a steady friend eventually pales in favor of being an anorexic or a bulimic. Sometimes, the eating disorder is so powerful that it becomes the only thing the person has in common with other people such as family, peers, friends and caregivers. It is always the topic of discussion, always the most important subject when they meet; it takes precedence over anything else they share. Although the eating disorder often brings negative atten-tion from others, it may be attention that was not there before—and it may not be there if the eating disorder ends.

Sometimes—particularly in a very sensitive, self-denying young person—the eating disorder brings attention to someone who has never before felt like the focus of attention. It allows someone to be "different" and allows people to show their concern—their love—through the mechanism of the eating disorder. It gives the dieter the feeling of being cher-ished and cared for, though in a very restricted and bizarre way. She may never have been a star athlete or child prodigy, but with the development of the eating disorder something exceptional has been gained. This is something she is better at than other people. Many times, others envy this control of eating and weight; "I wish I could have just a little anorexia," they may say. In this small aspect of life the anorexic can feel superior to them, and at some level she may even have con-tempt for others who do not have such incredible self-control and self-denial. All of these feelings are wrapped up in the anorexic's sense of identity as someone who "has the disease."

An emaciated person sends signals of illness to others, signals that something is not right. Many of us have a difficult time initiating relationships with unwell people, usually because we do not know what to say, and we may even feel uncomfortable around them. This allows the anorexic to isolate herself further. This isolation, though destructive, buffers the dieter from the rest of society, and prevents the constant interactions that, in her mind, may lead to failure. Some anorexics want to feel invisible; their goal is to feel small and insignificant so as not to be noticed, and dieting is used to accomplish this goal. Many people view the anorexic body as not attractively slim but quite unattractive, even hideous, and this usually eliminates any sexual signals. It certainly portrays the anorexic as being sexually unavailable, and this, of course, is a way for the anorexic to avoid sexual encounters, which could be another source of failure. In

Eating disorders and isolation

"Having an eating disorder is very isolating. I try to stay by myself and eat my own 'safe foods.' But I think it's more isolating to be bulimic than to be anorexic, and I've been both. When I first became bulimic I'd never heard of it. I thought I was the only person in the world who would do such a crazy thing. I felt totally alone in it. Currently I'm a restricting anorexic and bulimic. It makes it very uncomfortable and difficult to engage in eating affairs with other people, so I avoid them."

"Isolation is a close friend and yet it's also my foe. It keeps me insulated from the world, safe and comfy just to be with myself. However, I'm probably too isolated for my own good."

"I have very mixed feelings on isolation. It's comfortable yet it also holds me back in life. Sometimes it's extremely pleasurable, i.e., I couldn't care if I saw anyone in the world; sometimes it's a source of consternation, frustration, loneliness, sadness and pain and I want to escape from it and yet there's nowhere to go."

addition, the hormonal changes that starvation produces drastically eliminate the sexual drive. The combination of weight loss and hormonal changes produces an adult without any sexual interest or signals, an adult who has avoided, by her dieting, one of the most difficult, complicated and psychologically traumatic aspects of human life—that of forming close emotional and physical relationships.

Immediate Gratification

There is nothing like immediate gratification to make someone want to continue a behavior. The gambler who keeps making small gains with the expectation that the next card played or the next coin in a slot machine will pay off hugely, or the alcoholic who finds instant gratification with the next drink, thinks very little about the long-term consequences of these actions. In a similar manner, the mind-set of the anorexic or bulimic is reinforced by the immediate reward of dieting.

The loss of weight seen daily on the bathroom scales, the progressive emaciation seen in the mirror, the comments from friends and family, even the visits to physicians are, to some dieters, fairly immediate tangible rewards for their behavior. For some bulimics, eating large amounts of food at one time is a very unhappy urge to which they must submit, but purging brings immediate feelings of pleasure. They have rid themselves of the food, taking control of their hunger once again. They are tied up in the idea of control over these negative influences in their bodies. To see the vomitus come out and to "clean" themselves of the unwanted food is a positive, visible reward that perpetuates the behavior.

A Form of Personal Punishment

Coupled with the person's poor sense of self-esteem and perfectionism may be a desire to punish herself for her insufficiencies. Someone with an eating disorder often feels undeserving, useless, unwanted and worthless. She may feel that she is a "bad" person, and may be unable to understand why anyone else would be concerned that she has lost weight or that her eating is so abnormal, because she doesn't think she is worthy of the concern or love of family and friends. She feels that she is a burden to others, and she may be guilt-ridden because so many of their efforts are focused on her and she brings so much pain to those around her. Unfortunately this feeling of bringing pain and unhappiness to others (particularly friends and family) reinforces her feelings of low worth, and this is reflected in her trying to punish herself by perpetuating her eating disorder. She may say, "I don't deserve a better life," or "I'm not worth being healthy or respected." She may feel that, if she is very restrictive with herself with regard to eating—if she denies her own hunger and emotional needs severely—she will somehow atone for the pain and suffering she is causing others.

The Family and Eating Disorders

Is There a "Typical" Family?
Because many people first develop signs and symptoms of their eating disorder when they are young, the role of the family in the development of these disorders has been studied intensively in the search for some common feature or factors. Even the original accounts by Gull and Lasègue described the family as a hindrance to treatment. These physicians suggested that patients were better off away from family influence. Because the family is so important in the intellectual and emotional development of the young adult, it was suspected that in many cases the family environment somehow produced the disorder.

One group of studies in the late 1970s pointed to particular characteristics that were thought to apply to the "typical" family for the production of eating disorders. These investigators felt that lack of conflict resolution was a major problem; most family members avoided direct conflict and simply left difficult decisions unmade. This was referred to as "problem denying." The families were also felt to be overprotective of their young members. These investigators also noticed what they called "enmeshment," a lack of separation of the emotional needs of one individual in the family from those of the others. For some years these were understood to be the significant characteristics of a family that had children with eating disorders—the implication being that the family dynamics were somehow responsible. This was a cause of considerable anguish for many parents, who felt that their parenting methods were directly responsible for their children's eating disorders.

After further observation it is now understood that, in fact, this specific pattern of family dynamics is not frequently seen in families with children who have eating disorders. In one recent study the characteristics mentioned above are found in only one-fifth of the families. The understanding now is that eating disorders can arise in almost any type of family. There is no particular significance to the size of the family, the number of siblings, the birth order of the eating-disorder patient, whether it is a single-parent or two-parent family, or the mixture of sons and daughters.

It has been observed that there is more obesity and alcohol abuse in the families of bulimics, and that more open conflicts and major family problems are seen in the families of people with anorexia nervosa than in other families. There is no significant difference between the groups in the incidence of parental loss due to death or to breakup of the family. Childhood sexual abuse seems to be more common in anorexics; in one study 31 percent of anorexics had been abused sexually, whereas only 15 percent of the controls had been. ("Controls" are non-anorexics included for the purpose of comparison.)

Is the Family to Blame?

When you are faced with such a difficult problem as an eating disorder, it is human nature to search for some reason or cause. Because many eating-disorder patients are young, parents feel a personal responsibility for any illness that may occur in them. Often they blame themselves for the appearance and continuation of the problem that is having such a disastrous effect on their child.

However, most researchers now agree that, because there is no common family pattern, the concept of blame is irrelevant, and can be quite damaging. The current thinking is that these disorders occur because of a combination of genetic predisposition, emotional makeup and life experience. Many of these predisposing factors are not within the control of the parents. Many of the family characteristics that were proposed some years ago as possibly causing the disorders are in fact quite laudable and desirable. Such things as a close relationship among family members and the avoidance of direct conflict are not in themselves undesirable.

As soon as a family member develops an eating disorder, the family dynamics change considerably. The stress of a family member not eating properly is very powerful, and immediately changes the relationship among family members and the family as a unit. Many of the characteristics that were identified as being present in a "typical" family with eating disorders are characteristics that occur *as a result of the eating disorder*. Searching to assign blame, or blaming yourself, is not justified by the scientific facts. More important, it takes much-needed energy away from trying to deal with the disorder.

How Eating Disorders Change Families

Normal family routines are drastically disrupted by eating disorders. Events such as eating meals together, having family friends over, snacking in front of the television, going to restaurants, sharing special treats on special occasions, gathering for traditional holiday dinners and going on vacation are all affected. Frequently the person with the eating disorder refuses to eat with the rest of the family, or, if she does join them, mealtime is an uncomfortable time for everyone at the table. The person with the eating disorder feels she is being scrutinized and judged—"Like I'm a fish in an aquarium," says one woman—while the family becomes visibly upset that she is eating inappropriately. Often there is one meal for the anorexic and another for the rest of the family. Watching the anorexic or bulimic person not eat, or eat abnormally, is a painful experience for the rest of the family. Rather than being a chance for the family to enjoy each other, mealtime becomes a time of heightened conflict.

Eating away from home is even worse. Many of those with eating disorders feel acute emotional distress when they have to eat away from home, because they know that their behavior will be observed carefully by their friends or family. Anorexics feel that they will be forced to eat more than they are comfortable with, and that even then they will be subjected to pleading and lectures. Bulimics worry that if they eat normally they will have difficulty purging; they will not be able to find a convenient spot to vomit, and will be left with the hated food in their bodies. It's quite common for someone with an eating disorder simply to refuse to go to a restaurant, or to eat anywhere away from home. This keeps them away from social functions and further limits their social contacts.

Family trips and vacations become impossible. The person with the eating disorder can't handle the possibility that spe-

What happens to the family?

"The eating disorder confuses and alienates me and my family. It makes us argumentative and fills us with thoughts of guilt and blame."

"I'm presently not in contact with my family. However, in the past my 'fatness' has been commented on by them—not a lot, but I recall the situations, and feeling either embarrassment or indignation."

"My husband has left me because he can't deal with my eating disorder. My daughter worries about me because she doesn't think I'll live very long."

cific types of food may not be available on the trip. The fear of serious health problems if the individual is left behind—or is brought along—will often keep parents or other family members from going anywhere for extended periods of time. Anyway, it's just too emotionally taxing to carry all the eating-disorder issues experienced at home along on a holiday.

Relationships between family members become increasingly strained. Parents may disagree over how to deal with the anorexic or bulimic child, and treatment options such as therapy, medications and hospitalization bring out strong and sometimes opposing points of view as the parents try to deal with their sense of responsibility. Because the problem is not easily solved, it becomes a frustrating point of friction between family members who may not be able to agree on an approach. Parents may blame themselves, individually or collectively, or they may blame each other. One parent may feel rejected by the child while another feels alone in the care of the child, with all the responsibilities for decision-making falling on his or her shoulders. A parent may feel manipulated and even made a scapegoat while another parent is seen as the favored "protector."

The eating disorder becomes the dominant focus in family discussions and takes a great deal of energy. The parents are deprived of time that should be spent in strengthening their own relationship, and their relationship with their other children. Parents often feel very alone, vulnerable and unprepared to deal with such a significant illness. They may become obsessed with finding a cure for the eating disorder, and may spend much of their energy and time worrying about their child and trying to find adequate resources and solutions for a problem that appears insoluble. Often, they take an active role in trying to seek out help only to find that the child herself has no interest in being helped. Efforts to comfort, protect or care for the child often meet with disdain, yet deliberate attempts by the parents to become less involved may lead to such negative comments as "You don't care" or "You don't love me." Parents feel manipulated and confused in the light of the changing moods of their child. And because professional caregivers and literature about eating-disorder treatments give conflicting information, parents may feel there is nowhere to turn, no one to give them support and strength to carry on.

So much attention is given to the child with the eating disorder that siblings often feel left out or abandoned. They feel that their own normal needs are not being met, yet feel guilty for expecting attention under the circumstances. On the other hand, they may also feel protective and responsible for their sibling. All family members may feel that they have to "walk on eggshells" to avoid upsetting the member with the eating disorder, whose moods and behavior are quite unpredictable. They realize that she has a problem and needs their help, but nothing they try seems to make much difference.

Emotions and resentments build to extremes. Feelings of rage and anger emerge because the family feels helpless to make any change. The ordeal seems endless. Parents and siblings give up socializing with friends, going to concerts or parties, traveling, pursuing hobbies, education and career

Family dynamics that hinder recovery efforts

- a lack of communication
- hurtful, derogatory language between family members. Comments such as "You're not even trying to get better" or "You're just doing this for attention" only cause emotional pain, resentment and negative replies or an unwillingness to try to get better
- avoidance of obvious conflicts, which usually compounds the problem
- issues of control, which lead to power struggles
- ineffective problem-solving or coping strategies
- drug and alcohol use by any family member, which can make efforts to find resolution by others a formidable task
- denial that the eating disorder is a serious problem

opportunities, to try to deal with the problem at home. They feel that their lives revolve around the whim of the child with the eating disorder. Communication suffers (it doesn't seem to make much difference anyway) and family members stop talking to each other, and avoid each other in an effort to minimize confrontation and impasse. The entire family system circles in frustration, around and around.

What Can the Family Do?

There is no question that the family plays an important part in recovery. This process begins with open, honest, respectful and kind communication. If the family has used poor communication techniques, such as avoiding talking out problems, making unkind remarks to each other or walking away from conflicts, the members need to learn healthier communication. For example, a well-placed apology, when appropriate, can demonstrate a willingness to make positive change. Showing genuine concern and love for the person with the eating disorder is never inappropriate, and is simply a reflection of the deeply felt affection within the family.

Family members have to learn as much as they can about eating disorders, through either reading or external resources such as self-help groups, etc. A skilled family therapist may be able to allow each family member to have input into the altered dynamics of the family without directing blame at any one individual. Other support systems are also helpful in the recovery process. Parent or family support groups (facilitated by professionals) are helpful, as are the self-help groups (facilitated by parents of recovering individuals). These groups provide an opportunity for you to share your concerns, as well as to learn from others in a confidential environment. They also allow you as a family to see that there is hope for recovery, and to direct your energies toward the positive aspects of treatment.

Books focused on the family and eating disorders have valuable information. Family meetings, with or without the affected person present, offer a forum for discussion and for the ventilation of individual emotional responses. If you or other family members have substance addiction, you need a drug or alcohol treatment program. If you or other family members experience mental health problems, such as depression, manic-depressive illness or an eating disorder, treatment is also necessary. It is essential to maintain as normal a routine as possible, as a family and as individuals. Bring pleasurable or other meaningful events back into your life. Making the *family unit*—not the eating disorder—the valued entity is part of regaining control.

Dealing with a Family Member with an Eating Disorder

The eating-disorder sufferer herself is the only one who can make the decision to get help, and choose what kind of help she needs and wants. However, for your day-to-day relationship with her here are some suggestions:

- Try to avoid commenting on her appearance, even if asked directly. Your response is emotionally laden. Reply that you love her for the person she is, not for her weight or appearance.
- A simple expression of your affection is always appropriate. "I love you," "I care for you," "You are important to me"—these are all appropriate phrases at any time.
- Avoid direct conflicts around eating. Though it may be upsetting to you, the abnormal eating is simply a reflection of a more difficult and deeper problem that should be treated by therapy. Your indignation, anger or frustration should not show—your love should.
- Examine your own feelings about weight and shape, to be sure that you are not contributing to the importance the affected person places on these.
- Do not blame yourself for the problem.
- Do not blame the sufferer for the problem. These things occur of and by themselves; the sufferer did not choose for the disease to come, nor did she choose for it to take over her life.
- Learn as much as you can about eating disorders—from books, tapes, support groups and professionals.
- As in any illness, the sufferer needs your support but you are not her therapist. Focus on giving emotional support without condemnation or anger—showing your affection, building up her self-esteem and being available. Do not try to deny or minimize the problem, but do not try to be her therapist.
- Be optimistic. With the proper treatment and the passage of time there is every reason to believe that she will recover.
- Be patient. As much as you would like to, you cannot force the process to go faster than the pace she is comfortable with. Much of the frustration and anger in

dealing with eating disorders comes from impatience. It seems so obvious what should be done, but the sufferer doesn't seem able to do it.

• Be forgiving. Recovery will take time.

Advice to Parents

What do we do if we suspect an eating disorder is developing? First of all, don't panic. We can't help conjuring up the worst images we have seen in the media, but the fact that you are just beginning to suspect something suggests that an eating disorder, if it exists at all, may be in its early stages. There's time to collect your thoughts and find out the truth. Parents who show undue fear or even anger over the possibility of an eating disorder may send negative messages to their child. This will possibly make her want to keep her problem more of a secret, or make her feel she will not be supported by her own family—the exact opposite of what she needs.

One of the hardest tasks is to sort out what may be normal body image and diet trends of children or adolescents. Most of us go through periods of over-concern about how we look, how much we are eating and how much we weigh. The result is not usually an eating disorder. Keep this in mind before you conclude that there is a crisis.

If you suspect your child may be heading toward an eating disorder it is appropriate to confront her soon, to ensure that the problem doesn't continue any longer than it has to. Before approaching your child, think about whether she has been showing any undue concern over her weight or how she feels about her looks. Is she becoming depressed over her appearance? Does her behavior indicate that she is trying to do something about her body image, such as dieting, skipping meals or significantly increasing exercise? Do you suspect weight loss? Have you found laxatives or diet pills in her bedroom or elsewhere? Once you have pursued these possibilities, discuss your concerns with someone who will give you support and perspective. This may be your partner, friend or family doctor. Read books about eating disorders, including those directed at parents. You may want to talk to parent support groups, or professionals who have expertise with eating disorders, to get more helpful ideas.

When you do wish to share your concern with your child, find a quiet place to talk and be sure both of you, and anyone else involved in the conversation, have plenty of time. Present your concerns in a calm, respectful manner. Allow her to say what she wants, even if you know differently or suspect she is not being honest. If she agrees with what you suspect or know, find out why she feels she has to pursue weight loss. Is there peer pressure to lose weight? Is she in a competitive sport or dance classes where weight goals are stressed? Is she trying to be attractive to boys? Is she experiencing painful emotions that she is trying to control with her eating disorder?

If there is outright denial of an eating disorder, think about the comments she has used to defend her denial, and consider whether what she is saying may be true. If her explanations are credible, just keep observing her attitudes and behaviors to see where they lead. If you are still concerned, confront her again.

If you are sure there is an eating disorder, you will need to be persistent and have her see a counselor, and also have her see the family doctor for a medical assessment to rule out any impending health issues. If she refuses both options you may at least need to contact the school counselor or administration to inform them of your concerns; they may be able to limit her stress from schoolwork and extracurricular activities. Keep contact with support groups, friends and family while you go through this difficult period of your child refusing treatment.

Your efforts will pay off. Usually, children eventually face the fact that there is a problem. With all of your efforts to date you will be better prepared to face what is ahead, and to have supports in place to help you along the way.

Our child has an advanced eating disorder; what fresh approaches can we try?

If many treatment options have been attempted and there seems to be little headway, bring the treatment team together to discuss what has already been tried. Look at what has been successful and what hasn't. Approaches that have been helpful in the past may be useful again. Look at options not yet tried. Have you used all the resources available in your community? Are there caregivers using different approaches that seem plausible? Is treatment in another community an option? Have unresolved family issues or drug and alcohol issues been addressed adequately? Have you tried options mentioned in Chapter 9, "The Road to Recovery," including taking *time out* from treatment for now?

If a treatment plan is in place and the professional care-givers, as well as yourself, are confident that you are on the correct path, just continue the course—and give it more time!

How do we manage an eating disorder in a preteen?

Eating disorders are very rare before puberty. Before making an absolute diagnosis of an eating disorder in this age group it is important to rule out other causes of weight loss, loss of appetite or vomiting. Serious medical and emotional reasons must be considered before an eating disorder is diagnosed.

The health risks due to weight loss and dehydration to a preteen who does have an eating disorder are greater than to an older teenager or adult. Close medical monitoring is important.

How can we help a child away at college?

When a child with an eating disorder goes away to college, you may feel you are out of touch and not able to monitor her health. You can't give the personal support you are used to providing. Your child may be separating from her professional treatment programs and medical help, and may be left without treatment options in her new environment.

You can help by keeping in as close contact as is reasonably possible, through the telephone, e-mail or letters. Trips home for the child, or visits by the family, will help to keep family bonds intact. Find out what eating-disorders therapy and medical resources may be on campus or in her new community, and have these resources lined up ahead of time. There are often wait lists for these resources, and it could take months to access them. You will need to know what treatment options are covered by health insurance agencies, if indeed they are covered. If the distance and the cost of commuting aren't prohibitive, your child may need to return to her hometown for treatment already in place, even if it is infrequent. Caregivers in your hometown may also be able to keep in contact with your child through the telephone, e-mail or letters. If it is not essential that your child seek employment while she is at college, and if you can help her out financially, take the burden of work away and allow her to address her studies and, most important, give attention to the recovery process. Contact family friends or relatives near your child's campus, who may be able to give her support or even a place to stay.

If the child is becoming despondent, lonely and depressed, and the eating disorder is becoming worse, she may need to discontinue her classes for now and return home, where she has better support from family, friends and professionals.

How do we help a newly independent young adult?
Parents face a mixed set of emotions when an adult child with an eating disorder is leaving home. Her departure may bring a sense of relief. It may mark a milestone in her life that she has become mature and is breaking away from the state of arrested development that the eating disorder has perpetuated. It may indicate a real change in motivation for her to improve her eating disorder and create a life that is of her own making. Moving away may also relieve some of the stress that the family has been experiencing, and provide a reprieve for her and for other family members. On the other hand, leaving home may initiate more distressing feelings.

It may be that she wants to move away to avoid having to work on her eating disorder. There will be no one to monitor her eating behaviors or to watch for health risks. Moving out may mean that she will not have the financial means to live in adequate housing, and that she will have little money to buy food.

You can be helpful in many ways. You can keep in contact regularly. If you live in the same community as your child, visit each other as frequently as is practical and encouraged. Sometimes it is best to have less contact, when it only leads to arguments or regression in your child's eating disorder or moods. You may be able to provide financial support so that the burden of having to seek employment is lessened. Encourage your child to stay in close contact with her professional caregivers, or help her find new ones if she has moved to another community.

How do we explain this to other children?
Siblings are very intuitive about what is going on in their own home. All too often they are left out of involvement with the eating disorder. They tend to worry in silence, as they feel that

it is none of their business or that they don't want to worry anyone else when their sibling is the "sick one." They may even feel ignored by the rest of the family because so much attention is being focused on their unwell sibling, and harbor resentment over this.

Explain to them what the concerns are, without exposing them to too much detail about the eating disorder. Ask them what they think about what has been going on, and whether they are worried. Assure them that you and your partner, as well as the professional caregivers, are addressing the problem, and that they should not be overly worried. Ask them to come to you any time with any thoughts or worries they have. Make it clear that they are not responsible for "fixing" their sibling's eating disorder and that it is not their fault she developed it. Assure them that you love them but explain that it is necessary for you to spend more time with the other child until acute problems have been taken care of. Make a special effort to spend time with all your children on a regular basis, and keep family routines as normal as possible. Make sure the child with the eating disorder is involved in typical family activities as much as is practical. If one of the other children seem to be adopting eating-disorder attitudes and behaviors, give appropriate support immediately. Some siblings envy the attention their brother or sister is getting, or become seduced by the success of weight loss they have witnessed in their own home. Some may even want to compete with their sibling in weight loss. Family counseling may be useful to address the needs of everyone in the family, including the child with the eating disorder.

What can we say to friends and relatives? How can they help?
Eating disorders are very personal and you have a right to keep what goes on in your own family private. Not every-

one has to know. There are, however, times when it is necessary or even helpful to inform others of what the family is going through.

Determine who needs to know, and how much and what kind of information should be shared. If you are uncomfortable with letting others know about the eating disorder, but they have noticed something is going on, it may be enough to say, "My daughter is unwell but she is being taken care of. Thank you." If you need to give a more specific reason, you can say, "She has a metabolic problem" or "There is a concern about her stomach." People need not know more than you are comfortable revealing.

Sometimes friends and relatives must know about the eating disorder. Tell them just as much as they need to know, but enough to be helpful to you. Let them know about your emotional concerns and feel free to ask for their support. Let them know what treatment plans you have in place and assure them that it is not their responsibility to help treat the eating disorder. If they have helpful suggestions, accept this. If they seem meddling or interfere with your treatment options, distance yourself or ask them politely not to interfere. Give assurances that you are coping well, if this is the case, as they may worry needlessly.

Others can lend support in various ways. They may be available just to listen to you, over the phone or in person. They can help you "get things off your chest" and give you assurances. They may know of resources that you were not aware of or may be able to help you seek out support and treatment options. They may be able to care for your other children when you need to go to appointments or to the hospital. At times family or friends may be called upon to take your child, or even you yourself, into their home temporarily, to help relieve stress that may be tearing the family apart.

Some time away can do wonders for *all* family members. It allows space for all of you to settle your emotions and bring perspective to the situation. It's a safe, inexpensive way to bring peace within the family. It can be an important piece of the healing process.

Family support and eating disorders

"Eight years of my life have disappeared into the dark folds of anorexia and bulimia. I feel as confused by it as do my family and friends. I'm not incapable of rational thought—clearly I don't lack determination and drive, and I am not without ambition. I have a life blessed with an amazing family. Why me?

"My eating disorder gives me a sense of control, a place to rest my anxiety and obsessions—it makes all the decisions so I don't have to. I want to describe it as an entity, a force that hit me. My father calls it my "Ho Chi Minh," and I mostly feel helpless against such an enemy. It's really a slow suicide, not fully living and not fully dying.

"I experienced the truth of that a few months ago when I ended up in the hospital for my first serious crisis. I lay in a bed, hooked up to an I.V. and a cardiac machine. I was convinced I was going to die. The phrase "dead man walking" kept going through my head. I looked at my mother's face, and through her saw my brothers and my father too. These were people I wanted to get lost on a mountain with, and watch *The Simpsons* with. These were the people I would choose to be chained to. Nothing I had done had made them stop loving me. The possibility of great loss, greater than eight years to an eating disorder, became a tangible reality.

"I realized that none of this was a force that hit me after all. Ho Chi Minh was not an outside invader. Everything came from and was created inside me. I'm not a different person all of a sudden. Nothing became easy, but I began to see the fear, the anxiety and the eating disorder itself as an example of how powerful I could be, instead of how weak I could be. I'm using the very things that make me so sick to begin making me well.

"I don't understand it any more than I did three months ago, and don't care if I ever do. But I tattoo every glimpse of life in the forefront of my mind as reminders. I finally believe there is hope."

SIX

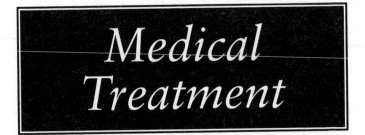

Medical Treatment

Alone in her darkened hospital room, lying in her bed, Shirley allowed herself to imagine what her life would be like without anorexia. The ward was quiet. The nurses had done their rounds for the evening and had dimmed the hall lights.

Shirley had been upset when her doctor first suggested that she come into hospital to get treatment for her anorexia. She saw it as a failure—just one more failure in a series of failures. She was afraid that she would have no control at all over what she ate or when she ate it. She thought she would be forced to eat food she couldn't stand, and would be subjected to endless counseling sessions with psychologists and psychiatrists, all of them thinking she was "crazy." She had felt much better when the doctor said that it was just for a short time, and that she would be allowed to participate in the decisions about her treatment—especially what she would be eating. Besides, she was quite worried about her potassium level. The doctor had told her that it was dangerously low. He had suggested that the hospital admission would be a good way to begin to recover from the eating disorder. It would allow her a change in routine, a change in environment, and intensive treatment. She wanted so much to get better that she had trusted him and allowed him to admit her. Now, as she lay in her bed waiting for sleep to come, she was glad.

The first days had been difficult: meeting with the nurses and other staff, agreeing on the details of her new diet with the dietitian and getting used to the ward routine. She was very frightened by the prospect of completely losing her anorexia. As strange as it seemed, she was afraid of what might be left behind when the anorexia was taken away. As the days passed she became more relaxed and self-confident as she began to recover. She could now see that the anorexia had taken over her life. She was putting on weight, but not so much that it frightened her. She still felt fat (especially in her legs), but she was able to eat three small meals a day without the anguish she had felt before admission.

It was exciting to think about leaving the hospital soon, returning home, completing her university studies and getting on with her life. She knew she wasn't cured; that would take much longer, with much more effort. But at least, with this admission, she felt she had begun to take back control of her life.

Eating disorders always alter the normal functioning of the body, through their abnormal patterns of nutrition intake. Sometimes these changes are minimal but often they are quite marked; the detrimental effects can be life-threatening. For example, restrictive anorexia nervosa decreases the amount and type of food eaten, and the body must learn to cope with the reduced quantity and variety of nutritive intake. Bulimia with binge eating presents the body with excessive food intake, and all this food is then forcibly evacuated, along with normal bodily fluids. The body tries to cope with this altered pattern of food intake and absorption. The more drastic the altered pattern of nutrition, the more the body has to strain to adapt to it. Human physiology is fairly adaptable, but there are limits to its ability to accommodate abnormal eating patterns. When these limits are exceeded, the medical complications become apparent.

The Importance of Medical Treatment

Because eating disorders are a complicated mix of physical and psychological abnormalities, successful treatment always includes treatment of psychological issues as well as restoration of a healthy diet. This treatment goal is usually achieved by a team of medical doctors, nurses, psychologists, nutritionists, social workers, physiotherapists and therapeutic exercise specialists. It is well recognized that the medical and physical consequences of the eating disorder can produce many of the psychological changes. Distorted attitudes and emotions can be caused and perpetuated simply by the altered eating pattern. In order to address the psychological aspects of the illnesses, it is first necessary to begin to reverse the physical abnormalities. Thus refeeding—supplying more food, and helping the person establish a healthier nutritional pattern—is a prerequisite for dealing with the psychological problems; psychological treatment by itself will not be successful. Much of our information concerning this interrelatedness of psychological and physical abnormalities is based on experimental starvation models, the most well known of which is called the Minnesota Experiment.

The Minnesota Experiment

In 1944, at the University of Minnesota, an experiment was carried out to determine the medical and psychological effects of starvation. At that time, American and other Allied forces were anticipating having to deal with the civilian survivors of mass famine in Europe—both concentration camp victims, and other citizens whose food supplies had been interrupted by war. Medical specialists wanted to learn more about the consequences of starvation. They designed an experiment to produce starvation and marked weight loss in volunteers, so that they could study the effects, both physical and psychological, of such starvation. The experiment is of great significance to the study of eating disorders, because it clearly demonstrates not only the marked physical changes that occur with starvation, but also the psychological abnormalities that occur, even in normal volunteers with no previous psychological problems.

In the experiment, 36 male volunteers (conscientious objectors who had chosen to participate in the experiment rather than be recruited as active soldiers) underwent a graded, progressive decrease in caloric intake over six months. After a control period of about a month (when their average intake was 3,500 calories daily), the men had their food intake decreased drastically, in order to produce a loss of about 25 percent of their ideal weight. During this period, the men received between 800 and 1,500 calories a day, in two meals consisting mainly of bread, potatoes, cereal, turnips and cabbages. (The meals were designed to mimic the diet that was prevalent in Europe at the time.) After this weight loss was achieved, the men were maintained on their lowered caloric intake for several months and underwent both medical and psychological studies. Next, they were allowed to increase their caloric intake under controlled circumstances, and studied again.

In the experiment, all of the physical changes that are seen in anorexia nervosa (including the formation of lanugo hairs, a drop in heart rate, blood pressure, muscle strength and bulk, swelling in the legs, intolerance of cold, etc.) were documented. In addition, many psychological changes were documented, simply as a consequence of the alteration in nutrition.

Psychological changes experimentally produced by starvation

- apathy, joylessness
- withdrawal
- depression and frustration
- decreased insight and will
- tiredness, mental fatigue, poor concentration
- moodiness and emotional instability
- obsessional behavior
- irritability, inability to sit still
- preoccupation with food
- loss of sense of humor
- hopelessness, fatalism
- negativism

The Psychological Changes of Starvation

The volunteers involved in the Minnesota Experiment were psychologically normal before volunteering. They had been carefully screened and found to have no ongoing behavioral or psychiatric symptoms. As the experiment proceeded many psychological symptoms appeared, and these were thought to be simply the result of changes in food consumption.

The men became apathetic and withdrawn. They reported that social interaction with others "was too much trouble" or was "too tiring." They became self-centered, manipulative and joyless and were uninterested in many of the activities and events that had given them pleasure before. They lost their sense of humor. They became irritable and frustrated, sometimes without any specific cause. They were unable to sustain any kind of mental activity or concentration. They became depressed, sometimes to the point of considering suicide. They demonstrated obsessional behavior, particularly with regard to their limited food intake, and complained of being sensitive to noise and to cold; they were nervous, indecisive and restless. They became negativistic, quarreled often among themselves and presented a pessimism and fatalism that they had not demonstrated before.

Much of their time, both awake and dreaming, was spent fixating on food. They talked about it often, imagined it frequently and dreamed about it nightly. Many of them changed their attitude to food completely—some who had not taken much interest in food before vowed that they would change their careers when they left the experiment, and become cooks, grocery store owners, butchers or other food handlers. They became obsessive about recipes, menus and food handling. The men would swap recipes. They were very sensitive to how frequently images of food appeared in films, books and newspapers. The specifics of food preparation and food types became the main topic of conversation and of daydreams. There was a marked increase in gum chewing and smoking as eating substitutes. All in all, their lives centered around the concept of food, and its relevance to them grew tremendously.

As a result of the Minnesota Experiment, scientists had solid evidence that marked psychological changes can occur in normal volunteers as a result of radically decreased food consumption. This is an important concept for beginning to understand eating disorders, because it demonstrates the interdependence of the physical and psychological abnormalities in these illnesses.

Those with eating disorders are not, of course, healthy volunteers in a starvation experiment. They have social and psychological stressors that helped trigger the syndrome. The Minnesota Experiment proved that continued inadequate nutrition (and subsequent weight loss) perpetuates and worsens the psychological problems that are present at the initiation of the disease. In addition, it emphasized the need to treat the physical abnormality (of low weight and poor nutrition) before beginning to deal with the psychological problems.

Eating disorders should be treated in hospital when there is

- severe or rapid weight loss
- severe medical complications of malnutrition (for example, low potassium, low blood sugar, fainting spells, chest pain, vomiting blood, irregular or severely low heart rate, etc.)
- significant suicidal risk or suicide attempts
- eating behavior or purging becoming out of control
- a chaotic, abusive or otherwise non-supportive home or family environment
- weakness so severe as to interfere with activities of daily living
- concurrent medical illness (such as diabetes mellitus)
- pregnancy
- concurrent escalating psychiatric illness (such as schizophrenia, bipolar affective disorder, etc.)
- failure of therapy outside of hospital

Refeeding in Hospital

By the time someone enters the hospital for treatment of an eating disorder, nutrition has usually become very poor. There may even be health risks that need to be closely monitored. The primary goal during some hospital stays is to help improve nutrition, as efforts at home have not been successful.

Sometimes just having the person come into hospital and receive support from staff is enough to improve eating. The nutritionist sits down with the person and works out different food options. A combination of normal foods and liquid food supplements is considered. (Liquid supplements are high-energy meal replacements with a good proportion of nutrients such as proteins, carbohydrates, lipids, minerals and vitamins.) From these food choices a daily meal plan can be created, which acts as a guide to nutrition. "Safe foods"—that is, foods the individual feels most comfortable (or least anxious) eating—are selected. Sometimes food brought in from home or a grocery store is used to boost the feeding process.

At times, however, improving nutrition in hospital is not as simple as this. The individual may not be motivated enough to want to eat, and may even resent being in the hospital. Trying to eat may create such anxiety and fear that these feelings paralyze the individual's efforts.

To deal with anxiety, medications that decrease anxiety and fear about eating are sometimes prescribed. Some of these medications are used to decrease anxiety throughout the day, and some are taken just prior to eating.

Some people cannot sit still, due to restlessness, or cannot stop exercising. Some are at medical risk and cannot afford to be physically active as they are so undernourished. In these cases a bed-rest plan may be helpful. One way of implementing bed rest is to set eating goals throughout the day. As an example, if the person is able to finish her small breakfast, she will be allowed to walk around the ward and do casual activities until the next meal or snack. If she is unable to finish her breakfast, she will be asked to stay in bed until her next eating time. Staying in bed allows her to conserve valuable energy and, at times, helps to curtail severe exercise compulsions. It also helps motivate the person to eat a bit more, so that she can be up and about after the next eating time.

If nutrition is not improved with the best efforts of the treatment team and the individual herself, and her health is failing, nutrition supplements may be delivered by nasogastric (NG) feeding. A liquid, similar to the liquid supplement discussed above, is fed into the stomach through a very thin, soft tube about the size of a thick spaghetti strand. The tube is inserted through the nose and swallowed into the stomach. The NG tube supplies a small but steady amount of nutrition 24 hours a day without the person having to eat more than is tolerable. NG feeding is never used to replace normal eating, but it helps improve nutrition when eating is progressing slowly.

Sometimes NG feeding is the fastest way to improve someone's nutrition so that she can leave the hospital. For school-aged children NG feeding may be used over the weekends only, so that they can stay home and attend their own school during the week. They must do their best, however, to eat at home during the week. NG feeding is *not* force-feeding—it is a lifesaving process that speeds the refeeding process and keeps hospital stays shorter.

When Does Hospitalization Become Involuntary?

If someone's nutrition has become poor enough to create life-threatening health risks or if she is at high risk of suicide, and she refuses to accept necessary treatment, it may be necessary to insist upon treatment in spite of her wishes. In these situations a legal certificate has to be signed by at least one and usually two physicians; laws vary from one region to another with regard to involuntary treatment.

Very few people require involuntary treatment, but having the process in place often stimulates a more concerted effort to accept treatment, even if grudgingly, and treatment may not actually be forced upon them. Often the individual who is starving is grateful that someone is taking responsibility for her eating, and that this dreaded burden has been taken off her shoulders. For someone who is suicidal, involuntary treatment provides safety measures to help prevent self-harm.

Types of Hospital Programs

Very few hospitals have eating-disorders programs. Of those that do, some have exclusively in-hospital programs while others have programs on hospital wards *and* in outpatient clinics where people can access treatment during the day or evenings while living at home.

Refeeding may be very successful even at a hospital that does not have a funded eating-disorders program, as long as the team members communicate with each other as well as with the person with the eating disorder.

Community-Based Eating-Disorders Programs
New eating-disorders programs tend to be separate from the hospital setting, especially for people who don't require hospital treatment. Community-based programs are generally less expensive and try to provide a less clinical environment. These programs may provide individual or group treatment for children, adolescents and adults. Some are specialized for a certain age group. If someone reaches the point of needing hospital treatment, her care may be continued in the hospital setting until she is healthy enough to return to the community-based program.

Normalizing Eating Patterns
The first goal of recovery is to begin to re-establish a healthy eating pattern. Often this must be done carefully, slowly and with individual attention, because the body has adapted to the abnormal eating pattern and is in a precarious balance. Any rapid change in eating can have a negative effect, such as worsening electrolyte and other biochemical abnormalities. Suddenly eating large amounts of food that have been avoided for months or years may cause abdominal pain and bloating. In addition, the psychological aspects of the illness often produce marked resistance to a rapid change in diet. Accordingly, the rule "start low, go slow" applies.

Refeeding programs can be established at home or in hospital, but a nutritionist usually supervises the refeeding. The nutritionist begins with a careful assessment of current nutritional intake and anticipated needs. Vitamin and mineral supplements and high-energy liquid drinks are often used at first, but the long-term aim is to use normal food to improve the nutritional status; this combats both nutritional inadequacy and psychological abnormality. The nutritionist usually suggests frequent small meals consisting of a variety of food choices, with snacks scheduled throughout the day. The person also needs support to re-establish mealtime as a time of social contact and pleasure. Activities after meals may be supervised to ensure that purging does not occur.

There is some debate as to whether the patient should be allowed to see her own weight regularly. Some therapists suggest that she should be allowed to see her weight on the scales because it gives a sense of control over her care, and may allay fears that the weight gain is too rapid. Others suggest that seeing the weight on a regular basis increases the patient's anxiety, especially when the weight is increasing, and interferes with progress. Each case should be decided individually. The ideal weight gain in hospital is between two and three pounds (about a kilo) per week. The person may expe-

Daily hunger patterns

The proportions of carbohydrates, proteins and lipids (fats and oils) in each meal or snack will affect how long it takes before the feeling of hunger begins again.

Meals or snacks consisting mainly of carbohydrates supply us with relatively fast energy. Carbohydrates can be either "simple" (sugary) or "complex" (starchy). Our blood sugar rises quickly if we eat the simple sugars found in desserts, candies and chocolate bars. Complex carbohydrates, found in foods such as breads, rice, potatoes and pasta, create a slower rise in blood sugar. After a carbohydrate meal, hunger will subside, but it can return within as little as one to two hours. People who eat mainly carbohydrates will be hungry frequently throughout the day.

To increase the time before hunger returns, it is best to add foods with proteins and lipids. The body takes longer to metabolize proteins and lipids, and so they suppress hunger for longer periods. As well, they provide valuable nutrition that carbohydrates cannot supply.

The meals in developed countries are typically breakfast, lunch and dinner, and the time between these meals is usually four to six hours. Since hunger will likely develop after two and a half to four hours, people often snack between meals. Snacks can decrease, to some degree, the amount of food eaten at mealtime.

rience abdominal bloating, early satiety, cramping or nausea, but these usually improve with time.

Common Medical Complications of Eating Disorders

The altered metabolism caused by eating disorders often produces a cascade of important physiological changes within the body, as the body tries to cope with its limited supply of energy through food. The specifics of the eating disorder are very important here—a binge eater who does not purge has a much lower risk of medical complications than someone with anorexia nervosa who maintains her low weight by purging. In general, the more restricted the diet and the more frequent the purging, the more stress is placed on the body's coping mechanisms, and the more likely medical complications become.

Though the list of medical complications is almost endless, here are some of the more common problems.

Cardiovascular

- hypotension (low blood pressure), causing fainting spells and dizziness
- decreased heart size (atrophy), causing diminished heart function
- irregular heartbeats and rhythm, causing palpitations and dizziness (can be fatal)
- heart failure, causing shortness of breath and weakness
- change in valve function (leakage of the mitral valve), causing a predisposition to lung congestion from heart failure
- markedly impaired response to the demands of exercise; diminished physical endurance, fatigue
- heart block (a failure of the normal electrical impulses in the heart), causing fainting, dizziness and weakness

Metabolic

- dehydration (abnormal loss of fluid), leading to fatigue, dizziness
- low body temperature (hypothermia), leading to a feeling of always being cold
- low blood sugar (hypoglycemia), leading to difficulties in concentrating or thinking, headache and fatigue
- altered blood chemistry, especially decreased potassium, phosphate, magnesium and calcium; these chemicals are essential for the normal functioning of the heart, brain and muscles, and alterations lead to many symptoms, such as weakness, palpitations, muscle cramping and fainting
- increased blood cholesterol, leading to an increased risk of heart attack and stroke

Renal (kidney)

- dehydration and altered blood chemistry (see above)
- kidney failure—inability of the kidneys to properly adjust the body's levels of water and essential nutrients and chemicals—which produces weakness, swelling and dizziness, and may be fatal
- swelling of legs, feet and hands due to fluid accumulation in these areas

Gastrointestinal

- swollen salivary glands, cavities in teeth and damage to gums (all from vomiting)
- delayed emptying of stomach, causing abdominal pain, bloating and vomiting
- constipation, often aggravated by abuse of laxatives
- decreased digestive enzyme secretion, leading to poor digestion of foods, causing abdominal pain, bloating and diarrhea

- altered liver metabolism (with increased liver enzymes), which may cause abdominal pain and/or jaundice
- irritable bowel syndrome (abdominal pain and diarrhea)

Musculoskeletal

- osteoporosis, a thinning of the bones due to insufficient calcium in the skeleton, which may lead to painful compression fractures, especially in the bones of the spine
- stress fractures, broken bones that result from overuse (such as excessive exercise) or osteoporosis, which weakens the bones, allowing them to crack or break
- muscle cramping, weakness and mechanical damage—such as stretching or tearing of muscles or ligaments (the tissues being weakened by inadequate nutrition)
- delayed growth in young people (inadequate nutrition stunts normal bone and muscle development)

Blood

- anemia (abnormally low level of red blood cells) leading to dizziness, weakness and fainting
- low white blood cell count and low platelets, leading to lowered resistance to infection and poor clotting ability
- decreased blood protein levels, leading to poor immunity and swelling of ankles

Neurological

- atrophy (thinning) of the brain, associated with impaired ability to reason or think properly
- epileptic seizures
- damage to peripheral nerves, resulting in numbness or altered motor function
- facial paralysis (Bell's palsy), leading to loss of movement of the muscles of the cheek and eyelids and mouth on one side of the face

Endocrine (hormonal)
- impaired insulin metabolism, causing either abnormally high or low blood sugar
- decreased estrogen (in women), causing the menstrual cycle to stop
- decreased testosterone (in men), causing loss of muscle tissue, weakness, shrinkage of testes and loss of sexual desire
- decreased thyroid hormone production, causing fatigue
- increased cortisone secretion, causing osteoporosis
- delayed puberty

Mai's Story

Even with hospital treatment, recovery can be a long, exasperating process. Mai's bingeing and purging had put her life at risk, yet her mind could not accept the dangers.

"I don't think I'll ever forget those endless days and nights in hospital. I cried myself to sleep at night, and awoke each morning to find a lab technician ready to take vial after vial of my blood. I dreaded the outcome of the tests as I knew poor results would mean another intravenous. Those IVs were worse than anything. Since I was so dehydrated, my body held onto any fluid it was given. I could literally see the water retention in my ankles, cheeks and hands the minute the needle was in. In my own mind I was a fat, bloated balloon. I couldn't even look at myself, I was so disgusted. I would stare at the ceiling while taking a shower, and I would wash quickly so I only briefly touched this "fat" that only I could see. The worst part was that I knew I was keeping myself in the hospital. I knew my blood tests would never improve if I kept sneaking down to the public washroom to vomit (the nurses locked my bathroom door after mealtimes). My doctors had been telling me for two years that my heart tracings were so bad that I could die from a heart attack at any time. My potassium level had been so low for so long that my kidneys were failing; I might need dialysis and a kidney transplant in a few years if I didn't stop this. But even after all these warnings, I had never thought anything serious would happen to me. Then one day I was found unconscious in a grocery store and taken to the hospital with cuts to my head. That was the first time I realized that something dangerous really could happen.

"Unfortunately I still feel a little that way. Not that I haven't made progress; I haven't been in hospital for over a year, which is a milestone. My heart tracings are normal and my kidneys are at much less risk of failing. My potassium is still a bit low, but it's better. I have my own apartment that I share with my three cats. When I was really ill I couldn't dream of holding even a part-time job; now I have *two* jobs. Unfortunately, most of my pay goes toward bingeing and vomiting. I'm still struggling with this part of my eating disorder. Having said that, though, I'm much happier today than I was a year ago. So maybe next year I'll be even happier."

Meal Support

One of the most challenging tasks of recovery, even with the strongest motivation, is increasing daily nutrition. Adding amounts and different kinds of food triggers anxiety and fear of body image and weight changes. For those who are used to vomiting or over-exercising after eating, they may find it very difficult to not use these ingrained (compensatory) behaviors.

One way to help someone cope with refeeding anxiety and fear is to provide meal support. Meal support occurs when others are available to eat with those with an eating disorder, and help to distract them during and after meals. Meal support can happen in the home, in a community eating disorders program or in a hospital. The supportive person may be a professional (nutritionist, therapist, nurse) or a family member or friend.

The supportive person can help by modeling healthy eating during meals and providing distraction after meals by taking the focus of conversation away from body image, weight or food topics. Anxiety can be lessened by having the supporter involve someone in grounding activities such as breathing exercises. Engaging in crafts, games or a movie after eating may help. After meals the supporter may discuss anxieties surrounding eating and highlight positive coping stratagies.

SEVEN

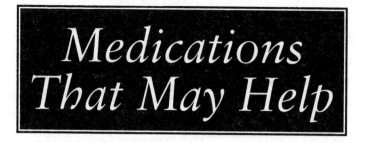

Medications That May Help

In the earlier part of the twentieth century, doctors believed that there was an endocrine (hormonal) cause for eating disorders, and treated them with various hormonal stimulants and supplements. These were the first "medicines" used to treat these disorders. It's now known that these medicines (such as thyroid extract and pituitary extract) are not effective.

In the 1950s and 1960s physicians used antidepressants and antipsychotic medicines to try to alleviate some of the psychological symptoms, such as depression. Antidepressant medications are still the medications most commonly used, but it is well accepted that they are almost never successful alone, because of the complex nature of these disorders. The best prospects for recovery are based on adequate nutrition and psychological therapy, sometimes accompanied by medications.

There is no one medication that has proven useful in all eating disorders. Someone with anorexia nervosa responds differently to medication than someone with bulimia nervosa or binge-eating disorder. Accordingly, the choice of drug, the schedule and dosage of drug use and the other particulars of the medications are decided by the individual physician and patient.

In the case of anorexia nervosa, when weight loss has been significant, treatment with medication alone will not make much of a difference. Many medications work by altering brain chemistry (particularly the neurotransmitters such as serotonin), and there is evidence that brain chemistry is already substantially altered in situations of malnutrition or starvation. Thus medicines will have little or no effect until the person begins to approach a normal eating pattern and his or her weight is rising. In short, the "drug of choice" in anorexia nervosa is food.

In many other eating disorders, a significant improvement can be achieved simply by restoring adequate nutrition and using some kind of psychological therapy (cognitive behavioral therapy, family therapy or a combination of both—see Chapter 8, "Psychological Treatment," for further details). Studies show that the use of medicines in these situations does improve the recovery rate, but only slightly. The main difference is in the incidence of relapse. A relapse is the return of an illness after partial or complete recovery. The relapse rate is much lower when medicines (particularly antidepressants) are used than when they are not used.

The comments below refer to drugs by their generic names. For examples of brand names, please see the drug table at the end of this book.

Drugs Commonly Used

Tricyclics
A class of drugs called *tricyclics* has been used successfully for decades to treat depression. Because of the common depressive symptoms seen in eating disorders (such as loss of joy in life, thoughts of suicide, deterioration in the quality of sleep and a sense of worthlessness or purposelessness), they

have been used to treat eating disorders. Tricyclics work by increasing the level of neurotransmitters (chemicals that act as messengers carrying information from cell to cell) within the brain. Examples of tricyclics include amitriptyline, nortriptyline, desipramine and imipramine. Common side effects include sedation and tiredness, dry mouth, constipation, low blood pressure, heartbeat irregularities and confusion.

Selective Serotonin Reuptake Inhibitors (SSRIs)

These drugs have been extensively studied in eating disorders, and fluoxetine, the first SSRI to be licensed for the treatment of depression, is the only one licensed for the treatment of bulimia. SSRIs work by adjusting the level of serotonin, a neurotransmitter within the brain. Serotonin levels have been shown to be associated with mood, and also with the feeling of being hungry or full. Drugs that increase the level of serotonin in the brain improve mood, and this group of drugs raises the level of serotonin by blocking the body's reuptake of that chemical once it is released, so that it stays effective longer. Examples of SSRIs include fluoxetine, paroxetine, sertaline, fluvoxamine and citaloprim. Venlafaxine, an antidepressant, related to the SSRIs, is becoming used more for depression as well as anxiety.

Fluoxetine is particularly helpful in the treatment of bulimia nervosa. In various trials, its use has been associated with a decrease in the number of binge and purge episodes, an improvement in general mood and a lessening of depressive symptoms. When continued for several months these drugs also reduce the chance of relapse. Side effects may include nausea, headache, agitation, reduced sexual desire, sleep disturbance and, paradoxically, decreased appetite.

It has been noted in several trials that the dosage of fluoxetine normally used to treat depression is not as effective in eating disorders as a larger one. For example, in one clinical trial involving 400 patients it was found that 60 mg of fluoxetine per day was clearly superior to a placebo, but 20 mg of fluoxetine per day (the usual adult dosage) was not. (A placebo is a non-active "fake" medication used for purposes of comparison.) Because of this difference, some experts believe that when fluoxetine is used for bulimia nervosa it does something more than simply treat the depressive aspect of the disease.

Anxiolytics

Anxiety is a feeling of being uneasy, worried, agitated or excessively concerned about an imminent danger or difficulty. It is a protective mechanism that allows us to anticipate problems in our environment so that we can begin to prepare ourselves for them. Anxiety is a prominent symptom in many people with eating disorders, particularly as they begin to normalize their nutrition. Sometimes the anxiety is bad enough that it needs to be treated. The drugs used to treat anxiety are called anxiolytics.

The most common anxiolytics used belong to a class of drugs called benzodiazepines, and this group includes such drugs as lorazepam, diazepam, oxazepam, flurazepam, clonazepam and others. All the benzodiazepines have the same result: a calming sensation or quietening of anxiety, caused by the chemical's effect on the transmission of nerve signals. The big difference between benzodiazepine compounds is the length of time that they act in the body. "Half-life" is the name given to the time it takes to break down half the drug in the bloodstream: the longer the half-life, the longer the drug's effects. These drugs are often used to calm fears about refeeding and to allay anxiety, and are sometimes used to help with sleep. Side effects include excessive drowsiness and confusion, inability to think clearly and forgetfulness. Tolerance to these medicines develops quickly, meaning that the drug becomes less effective and it may be necessary to increase the dosage. Frequent use sometimes causes "rebound" anxiety when the drug is stopped.

Appetite Suppressant and Enhancing Agents

Many medications have been studied for their ability to either suppress or enhance appetite. Although there have been some successes in controlled situations with "normal" people, follow-up studies have not proven these drugs useful for people with eating disorders. Fenfluramine increases the serotonin level by blocking its reuptake and enhancing the neurotransmitter's release within the brain. Early studies produced encouraging evidence of appetite suppression, but subsequent trials have not shown that this drug is helpful. Because fenfluramine has been shown to have a severe effect on the heart valves of some people, it is no longer available.

It was noted in the 1960s that cyproheptadine, a serotonin and histamine antagonist (an antagonist is a drug that blocks the effect of another chemical), caused weight gain by stimulating appetite, but this effect is seen only in healthy people, not in those suffering from anorexia nervosa.

Human growth is regulated by a pituitary hormone called growth hormone. Growth-hormone releasing factor has been used in limited studies to stimulate the release of growth hormone, in an effort to stimulate weight gain, but it is not widely used.

Gastrointestinal Drugs

People with eating disorders, particularly those with anorexia nervosa, complain of early fullness, vomiting, constipation and bloating, especially during refeeding. Their stomach muscle contractions (peristalsis) are abnormal, and food often remains in the stomach for some time before being passed on to the small bowel. Agents such as metoclopramide, domperidone and cisapride have all been used to improve peristalsis and gastric emptying and thus relieve the symptoms of bloating and abdominal distress. Cisapride has been shown to cause sudden cardiac death and is no longer available. Rectal suppositories or enemas may be useful for constipation. Stool softeners, which are not laxatives, help keep bowel movements regular.

Drugs for Osteoporosis

Many eating-disorder patients (especially those with anorexia nervosa) develop osteoporosis—a marked thinning and softening of the bones due to a decreased concentration of

The treatment of eating disorders

Anorexia nervosa
- The condition does not respond to medicines alone.
- The "drug of choice" is food.
- Fluoxetine (or other SSRI antidepressants) may be used to relieve depressive or obsessional symptoms.
- Anxiety-relieving drugs are often used during the refeeding process.
- Gastrointestinal drugs are often used to relieve abdominal distress during refeeding.

Bulimia nervosa
- The condition can often be treated without the use of medicines.
- Fluoxetine has been shown to be effective when combined with psychological treatments.
- Anxiety-relieving drugs can be used for short periods.

Binge-eating disorder
- The condition may be treated successfully without the use of medications.
- Antidepressants reduce the frequency of binge-eating episodes, as well as depressive symptoms and the preoccupation with food.
- Without ongoing psychotherapy, drug therapy usually ends in relapse.

calcium—because of a combination of poor dietary intake, low blood-estrogen levels (in women) and high blood-cortisol levels. However, clinical trials have shown that estrogen supplementation alone (such as the birth control pill) does not improve osteoporosis in women, nor does simply treating them with calcium and vitamin D. The best results are obtained by refeeding and establishing a more normal nutrition pattern; this allows the woman herself to begin to secrete estrogen again, and to reverse the osteoporosis. Nevertheless, adequate calcium and vitamin D intake and estrogen replacement are used to minimize the osteoporosis.

A Promising Medication

Olanzapine is a medication that has shown some effectiveness in the treatment of anorexia nervosa. It seems to help decrease anxiety associated with eating, in part, by decreasing body image and weight concerns often associated with refeeding. This allows some with anorexia nervosa to improve nutrition and to gain weight. Further studies of this medication are needed to determine its overall effectiveness.

EIGHT

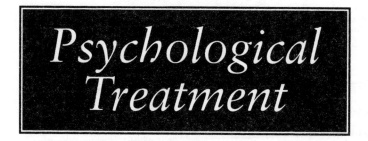

Psychological Treatment

The word "therapy" comes from the Greek *therapeia,* "healing, nurturing, tending in sickness." "Therapy" is a general term. It can refer to the work of a professional therapist with someone who has a health problem. It can also refer to healing continued on your own with guidance from a professional. Therapy can also be done entirely by yourself, with the help of books or techniques learned from therapists or therapy groups.

Therapies for Eating Disorders

Many kinds of therapies have proven useful: physiotherapy, occupational therapy, massage therapy, drug therapy, and many kinds of psychotherapy.

Psychotherapy refers to the treatment of disease or illness by psychological means. The word is a shortened form of "psychological therapy," meaning therapy that addresses mental (thinking and memory) and emotional concerns. Professor Arthur Crisp, an eating-disorders specialist from London, England, describes psychotherapy as "change through communication." Psychological therapies include cognitive behavioral therapy, art and music therapy, family therapy, interpersonal psychotherapy and many others. In the treatment of eating disorders, physical therapies, chemical or drug therapy (medications), and psychological therapies may be used individually or in combination.

What Makes Therapy Work?

Although there are hundreds of kinds of psychological therapies, only a few have been adapted for use in the treatment of eating disorders. Some have been proven to be very effective but, as with any treatment for any health problem, the same approach may not be effective for everyone. The book *Escape from Babel* (see Further Resources, at the end of this book) identifies four common components of successful therapy. These are extratherapeutic factors, the therapeutic relationship, the therapeutic techniques, and hope and expectation that the therapy will work.

Extratherapeutic Factors

Much of the success during a period of therapy happens outside the formal boundaries of the therapy. It takes all kinds of strengths for you to have made it through life to this point. These same strengths can help you deal with the eating disorder. Your therapist can help you identify other personal strengths. Think of all the life challenges you have faced already, and appreciate the great skills and resources you have had to rely on to deal with them.

Environmental factors also affect you. These include the people in your life—family, friends, co-workers, classmates and others. When we are troubled by life events, those around us can have a significant influence on our recovery by helping us to deal with our difficulties. Our living, working and school environments have an impact on us as well, and can help bring positive change.

There are also chance happenings. Often the most significant positive changes in our lives "just happen." Many positive experiences, such as new personal relationships, job options or educational opportunities, happen more or less by sheer luck.

The Therapeutic Relationship

The therapeutic relationship is the relationship that exists between the therapist and you. A number of factors contribute to form a positive therapeutic relationship. The therapist must be seen as empathetic, respectful and genuine. He or she must express warmth, and be trustworthy and nonjudgmental. The therapist does not tell you what to do, but acts as a co-worker or copilot in your treatment. The therapist must be a good listener, and must be able to express understanding and find ways to help you help yourself.

Therapeutic Techniques

The task of the therapist, aside from helping you to identify difficulties and problems in your life, is to show you possibilities for bringing about positive change. He or she can help you identify your emotions, face fears, take risks and alter old patterns of behavior. These tasks can be accomplished, in part, by various techniques that are part of each therapeutic approach.

Hope and Expectation

Therapy should, at the very least, provide an element of hope. The expectation that there is a way out of the eating-disorder maze can go a long way to bolster your optimism. You need a reason to recover, and the promise of realistic avenues to a better life. The therapist or therapy group should help validate your strengths, and should nurture these strengths. Elements of positive change need to be supported and encouraged. Therapy will help to raise possibilities and treatment options.

Watch out for quackery

Any health problem that is difficult to treat is an invitation to quack practitioners. Because established treatment options may have failed or are not available, people become desperate to make things right. They become prey to quackery.

Quacks take advantage of the despair and frustration you are going through. They assure you that other professionals can't help, and provide false hope that they are the only ones who can. They *promise* cure, a temptation no one wants to be denied. They claim to be "professionals" but often have few or no qualifications. They are not part of any mainstream health-care system, but say they have been rejected by other professionals because of jealousy over their success where others have failed.

Quack caregivers often do not belong to any professional colleges that set standards of competence. They are not accountable to anybody for their treatment practices. They are likely to quote well-known people as "expert" testimony to their abilities, and may parade indebted parents and patients as evidence of their success.

Guilt is a powerful weapon of the quack, who may shame parents into spending a lot of money on questionable care by making comments like "Do you want your daughter to die?" or "Don't you care enough?" People sometimes spend hundreds of thousands of dollars on treatment, and some sell their homes and other personal assets to meet payment. Note that the quack may provide treatment "for free" initially, to gain the family's trust, and ask for money later. Sometimes treatment is provided for free or for a discount, and later the family is asked to go to the press to state how exceptional the care has been. Some people have even had to work off their "debt" in the quack treatment facility.

Quack treatment programs are rife with emotional, physical and sexual abuse. Be sure you know what you are getting into before you commit yourself, your loved one or your wallet.

What Do Therapists Do?

If psychotherapy can be described as change through communication, the therapist can be defined as a catalyst for change. (A catalyst is something that allows a change to occur without itself changing.) Therapists allow you to see that change is possible, and they help you make that change.

Therapists have different functions, depending on whom they work with and the therapeutic tasks they undertake.

They can help identify the problems you are facing. They may diagnose specific health issues and suggest solutions to problems. As an example, they can be helpful in judging whether there is an eating disorder and, if so, what kind of eating disorder it is. They may be able to diagnose other health concerns such as depression or anxiety. They may pinpoint stresses in your life, such as harmful personal relationships or destructive life situations. They can help point out unhealthy thinking processes that lead you to repeated, inappropriate behaviors. They may assist you in recognizing factors that trigger negative attitudes and harmful behaviors.

Therapists can also be helpful just by listening to you and validating your feelings and experiences. They can act as mentors and role models, and often bring a lifetime of personal experience along with their training. They can help you focus your energies in positive directions, and they can stimulate optimism and hope. They can help you believe in yourself, and raise possibilities for finding constructive solutions to your life challenges.

How Does Therapy Change Anything?

All of us have experiences in life that help to shape the way we think and subsequently behave or act. Most of the time our actions or behaviors are rational, appropriate and responsible, but people who have eating disorders often have illogical thoughts that lead to inappropriate behaviors.

An example of an illogical thought is "If I lose weight, people will like me more." This thought originates in an irrational fear that you will not be liked if you are not thin. The inappropriate behavior in response to this is starving yourself or vomiting to lose weight. We often don't recognize these irrational thoughts—we may act in response to them without perceiving the origins of our actions. That's why we need a

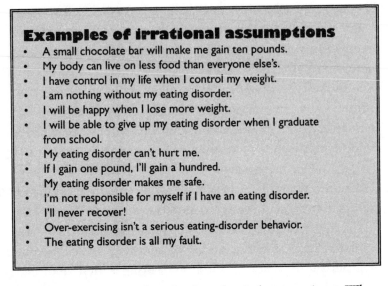

Examples of irrational assumptions
- A small chocolate bar will make me gain ten pounds.
- My body can live on less food than everyone else's.
- I have control in my life when I control my weight.
- I am nothing without my eating disorder.
- I will be happy when I lose more weight.
- I will be able to give up my eating disorder when I graduate from school.
- My eating disorder can't hurt me.
- If I gain one pound, I'll gain a hundred.
- My eating disorder makes me safe.
- I'm not responsible for myself if I have an eating disorder.
- I'll never recover!
- Over-exercising isn't a serious eating-disorder behavior.
- The eating disorder is all my fault.

therapist to help us identify these buried perceptions. When you are recovering from an eating disorder, it is important to identify your irrational thoughts and fears, and then work on adopting more positive, realistic thoughts. Once healthier thoughts are realized, you have a chance to change your destructive eating-disorder behaviors.

What Kinds of Therapy Are Used?

One of the commonest forms of psychological therapy in the field of eating disorders, dealing with changing what we think in order to change our behaviors, is cognitive behavioral therapy (CBT). It was first adapted for eating disorders by Dr. Christopher Fairburn of Oxford, England. "Cognitive" refers to the mental faculties of perception and reason; these include internal and external influences that create thoughts and visual images—how and what we think. The "cognitive" aspects addressed in treating eating disorders are extreme concern about shape and weight, perfectionism and all-or-nothing thinking, and low self-esteem. The "behavioral" component tackles disturbed eating and purging habits. Education and goal-setting, through working with therapists or groups, using reading materials and doing homework assignments, are all part of CBT.

Another form of psychological therapy, interpersonal psychotherapy, addresses some of the poor interactions people have with others, which can lead to repeated inappropriate behaviors. It does not work as quickly as CBT but it has a similar long-term effect.

Whatever therapy is being used, nutrition education and counseling seem to make a significant improvement in the final result.

Many other therapeutic approaches have been tried and may well be helpful in specific cases, but they need further long-term study to help determine their effectiveness.

Individual Therapy or Group Therapy?

Group therapy offers some advantages over individual therapy. It is usually more cost-effective than individual therapy, as it allows fewer staff to deliver treatment to more patients. Group therapy also allows you to meet others who are experiencing the same things. It may be the first time you have met someone who shares your thoughts, emotions and behaviors, and can understand and not be judgmental. It can help you feel that you are not alone.

Individual therapy is most useful when there is urgency or a crisis. It is also used exclusively for children and young adolescents, who typically avoid group situations and often do not work well in groups. People with anorexia nervosa tend to respond to individual therapy and not to group therapy.

Family Therapy

Eating disorders have a profound effect on families. While these disorders can help bring families together, they always cause some level of distress. Stresses can cause a breakdown of the whole family unit if there isn't some form of intervention.

Family therapy is helpful in bringing the family together to provide better support for the member with the eating disorder, as well as the rest of the family. The family therapist allows family members to express their frustrations as well as their heartfelt love for each other. Family miscommunication, which leads to misunderstandings, is addressed, and positive solutions are explored. The therapist identifies strengths within the family—strengths that are key to keeping the family intact. Family sessions may also identify factors that hinder progress, such as drug and alcohol use, or violence by family members.

Family therapy is not about assigning blame. It aims at finding rewarding solutions to help the healing process for everyone in the family.

Art Therapy

People with eating disorders tend to keep their emotions well guarded, and to avoid emotional contact. They are good at blocking any attempts to contact their inner world. They often become harsh critics of themselves, suppressing their needs and emotions.

Verbal therapy tends to arouse their defenses and prevent progress, but art therapy allows the person to keep communication open with herself and her therapist. Where verbal therapy may be threatening, due to the emotional pain involved, art therapy is often a "safe" way to express difficult emotions—sometimes unknowingly.

Art therapy may be useful in dealing with body image and weight fears, anxiety surrounding eating, and the distorted family dynamics created by an eating disorder. It can also identify issues not related specifically to the eating disorder—for example, emotional distress over the parents' divorce.

Different art media are used, including paints, pastels, collages and cutout figures, and clay. Clay allows an image to be expressed in three dimensions—a more realistic and tangible expression of the human body, and a useful tool when dealing with body image.

Occupational Therapy

Occupational therapy (OT) provides a number of useful skills and activities for people with eating disorders. The therapist helps them learn different coping mechanisms for dealing with their eating disorder. They learn to plan their day, making time for meal support (having someone sit with them during and after eating), for food shopping, for relaxation techniques to help them relax before and after eating, and for moderate exercise, when appropriate.

The person also learns what activities can be modified to conserve energy. As an example, exercise that burns up too much valuable energy may be replaced by activities such as reading, crafts or yoga. The therapist suggests maximum amounts of exercise, based on the person's state of nutrition, explaining what normal exercise is, and how over-exercising affects health.

OT helps people sort out what is important to do in a day and what is not. Quality-of-life activities that do not focus on eating-disorder treatment are an important part of therapy. These are activities that make a person feel better about herself, such as meeting with friends who support each other in positive ways. OT also helps people learn to be more assertive.

Relaxation techniques encouraged are deep breathing, yoga, visualizations, imagery, progressive muscle relaxation (where groups of muscles are first tightened, then relaxed) and autogenics (a technique of imagining parts of the body as they relax). Music and recorded sounds of nature (waves and birds) are also used.

For older adolescents and young adults there is emphasis on practical aspects such as taking vocational aptitude tests, writing résumés and dealing with interviews.

Stopping Techniques

All too often those with eating disorders worry excessively about body image, weight and food, as well as other issues (school, family, career). Some worry helps us to pay attention to the things in our life that are important, but it is often excessive and only creates more problems. Over-worrying can make the eating disorder worse, cause poor sleep and make individuals depressed and anxious. It can aggravate drug and alcohol abuse.

Stopping techniques are methods of interfering with negative repetitive thoughts (thought stopping) and unwanted behaviors. They help to take us out of our obsessive mind frame (worry) or destructive behaviors (bingeing, purging).

Stopping techniques include visualizing a big red and white stop sign, yelling "Stop" out loud or snapping an elastic band worn on your wrist. These can allow a brief time for you to refocus thoughts or behaviors onto healthier ones. Healthier thoughts may include imagining a special place or future planned event, and healthier behaviors may include relaxation techniques, including yoga or meditation. See sidebar on page 181 "Things you can do to help avoid a binge."

Stopping techniques can work very well but must be practiced daily, sometimes for a few weeks, before they become immediate and routinely successful. The more you practice them, the less negative thoughts and behaviors will be a problem.

NINE

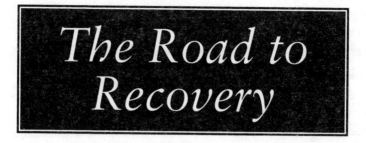

The Road to Recovery

Gayle's horror story began 13 years ago, when she discovered her younger daughter, Caroline, making herself vomit. At the time, Gayle and her husband, Ted, knew very little about eating disorders. They tried to find reasons for their daughter's anorexia, and a plan of treatment, but they couldn't find enough information in their small community. Deeply distressed, they searched the library, and finally tracked down a doctor in a nearby city who could give them some help. Caroline had two lengthy stays in hospital, but came out even more entrenched in her behaviors. Gayle and Ted didn't know how to handle the problem. Today—so many years later—they still aren't sure how to support their daughter without supporting her anorexia as well.

"Caroline ate from four p.m. to seven p.m. daily," Gayle explains. "But if we had company she wouldn't eat for that whole 24-hour period—not until four the next afternoon. We didn't want her to go without food, so we gave up having people over. But we needed our friends—obsessive-compulsive behavior and laxative abuse were new to us, and we were desperate. We really felt the social isolation, we felt alone in our struggle.

"Family therapy helped, but only for a little while. Ted was very angry—upset that he couldn't fix this problem. Our older daughter felt she had lost her parents' attention, as well as her sister, so she was angry too. I was swamped, trying to cope with everyone else's feelings, and a sick child, and my own anger and guilt.

"Eight years ago Ted retired and we all moved to the west coast. There we found an eating-disorders organization, a family service organization that provided therapy. What a boost of hope—a real lifeline! We gained some understanding—that this disease was not our fault, that it was our daughter's responsibility to change, but that family dynamics do contribute to the course of the disorder. Boy, we were happy to gain this new insight, and Caroline made some psychological progress. But then she turned 19 and she was dropped from the program; it was only available up to age 18. For a while the only therapy we could find was costly private counseling. This falling through the bureaucratic cracks was a whole new frustration to deal with.

"We found an adult eating-disorders program that admitted her for a while, but then they told us, 'Deal with this in your own community—we don't have space right now.' But our local hospital has no protocol on how to handle eating disorders. More frustration and anger. The local hospital did treat her for dehydration, and admitted her for refeeding when it was necessary, but no specific psychological help was provided for the eating disorder.

"Finally we found a great parents' support group. We had to fight a little to get into it, as it's outside our district, but it has provided us with a safe haven for unloading our feelings, including guilt. The group members aren't judgmental. Their attitude is 'Been there—done that.' They understand, and they've saved my sanity!

"Our greatest fear of losing Caroline came three months ago. At her lowest weight ever, and with her potassium level so low that cardiac arrest was a real possibility, she was put in the intensive care unit for ten days. She survived, and at last we're seeing an attitude change. This is great! She's still in hospital but she's healthier now, although she's far from well. She struggles every day. We encourage her to search her spiritual side and rely more on God's help. He will not let her down. He'll always love her and care for her. Our family is continuing its struggle for understanding, and we're gradually getting better facilities for our daughter and others who suffer this terrible problem. Bureaucracy moves slowly, but we want our struggle for Caroline to help other people too.

"We remain optimistic. We see small signs of change and progress, and we keep fighting for our child. We continue to hope and pray for her recovery. This beautiful, loving, intelligent person has so much to offer the world. We can't give up. We can't let the anorexia win."

What is recovery? How do I get there? When will I know I have recovered? These are questions often asked by those affected by eating disorders. The road to recovery includes many challenges and opportunities, but one thing is certain: it is yours to travel if you wish. Although it takes a lot of commitment and hard work, most people with eating disorders do recover. Once you understand what to expect along the way to recovery, the journey becomes easier.

What Is Recovery?

As you begin this journey, you should have a clear idea in your mind of your goal. What is recovery? You will have recovered when you can say, "I no longer have an eating disorder." This will mean that you have regained control over your own eating, body

What is recovery?

"Recovery is something I will probably never attain. I know that sounds like a defeatist attitude, and people might say, 'Well, if you're never expecting to get better, why keep going to doctors?' I have to keep trying. I have to keep hoping. Maybe someday something will click. I can't just let myself go. I guess I can say I'm 'in recovery' though not recovered."

"It's a process of self-healing, self-discovery, openness, willingness, awareness, trust in self, commitment and recommitment, allowance for setbacks, persistence, risk-taking, feeling feelings, self-affirmation, sharing with others, acceptance at each emotional, physical, spiritual level."

"Recovery is having my needs met without hurting others. It is feeling my full strength."

image and weight concerns. Eating-disorder attitudes and behaviors will no longer be a significant factor in your life. You, not the eating disorder, will be directing your life. This does not mean that you will never think of food and eating again. Some people who have recovered say, "I still occasionally think that I could lose a few pounds, or that I have eaten more than I should have." But these are now the thoughts of an average, healthy person. The difference is that you will have these thoughts for brief periods of time, and will not let starvation, vomiting or other eating-disorder behaviors take over because of these feelings. Moments of self-doubt and insecurity are normal for all of us. Recovery means that, instead of using eating-disorder behaviors to cope with such feelings, you will be able to use constructive techniques to make your way past them. When you have regained possession of your life and you can live happily without the eating disorder, you will have recovered.

Who Recovers?

One of the myths about eating disorders is that they are incurable. With very few exceptions, anyone with an eating disorder can improve his or her life and expect recovery. Even those whose eating disorders seem to have lasted years often find that, with the right support, their quality of life and general health can be greatly improved.

Am I Ready to Begin?

This may seem like an odd question, but beginning the journey to recovery demands a commitment, a realization that life with the eating disorder is no longer acceptable. You have to want to move, with all your energy and resolve, toward a better life. This readiness to recover may be a conscious decision, or it may come to you as a spontaneous awareness. Simply reading this chapter indicates that you are considering the possibility of changing toward a better life. The optimism that there is a better life waiting for you allows you to begin making that change.

Sometimes, a major crisis—loss of support of loved ones, hospitalization, a career loss or a significant threat to health—brings someone to the point of accepting recovery as an option. Sometimes, without any such major loss or change, a sense of enlightenment presents recovery as a possibility. Often, during treatment, someone begins to understand the pattern of illness and abnormal thinking, and starts considering the changes that would favor recovery. It's as if a series of lights were being turned on, signaling what has been obvious to others. It's as if you say to yourself, "Ah-hah, now I get it," as you begin to comprehend what the eating disorder has done to you. When this happens, you will begin to aim for something better. You will be ready to begin the process of recovery.

What Is the Path to Recovery Like?

Recovery from any emotional or physical health problem is never immediate. No matter how simple the problem, there is always some period of time that must pass before the state of recovery can be reached. Often, the more complicated the problem, the more time must pass for the changes to take effect. Recovery from an eating disorder is no different. It takes lots of time and effort, and the process resembles any other pathway; as you travel along it, things happen. You meet challenges you must overcome, and problems to which you must find your own best solutions.

Unlike many medical problems, such as asthma, acne or tonsillitis, in which a standard treatment works for most people, eating disorders are highly individual. There is no "standard" treatment, which is one reason why recovery can take such a long time and demand such a lot of energy.

There are often several variables involved. One is the abnormal eating pattern itself. Most people with an eating disorder use two or more behaviors to maintain their disordered eating—while one person uses fasting and laxatives, another may use restricting and vomiting. In addition, there are individual issues such as attitudes toward weight and body image, and factors such as depression, obsessive-compulsive traits and personality disorders. Your combination of all these variables produces your own pattern of disordered eating. Your path to recovery must be tailor-made for you.

The path is not a straight line. Sometimes it's hard to tell that you're making progress because, as you attempt to improve one behavior, another temporarily becomes worse. For example, if you're trying to decrease the number of times you vomit in one day, you may find that you compensate by increasing your exercise or more severely restricting your food. You may, in fact, feel that you are getting worse. In this situation, it's important to step back and evaluate what your eating disorder was like earlier. Over a longer time period, such as six months or a year, improvements in one or two variables may be clearer. You may have been bingeing and vomiting five

Things you can do to help prevent vomiting

- Set a time of 15, 30, 45 or 60 minutes during which you will not vomit after eating. This waiting time may help the strong drive to vomit pass. If you feel you have to vomit after that period, you still have the choice of doing so.
- Have someone stay with you during and immediately after eating.
- Pre-record television shows, and watch them when you need the distraction.
- Go for a walk; better yet, take a dog for a walk.
- Talk to someone on the telephone.
- Leave the bathroom door open when others are around.
- Take medications that help to decrease bingeing and purging.
- Do not buy foods that lead to bingeing.
- In your bathroom, tape up a list of health problems that vomiting can cause.

times a day, taking laxatives, over-exercising two hours a day, fainting regularly and feeling severely depressed. You may have been in the hospital. You may have been failing at school or not able to hold a job. Today, six months later, you may still be bingeing and vomiting but only once a day. You're not taking any laxatives, you haven't fainted for months, the hospital time is a distant memory and you're holding down a part-time job! Yes, you still have bulimia—but by sitting back and looking at the progress you've made, you can assure yourself that you are well on the road to recovery.

One of the earliest signs of progress is a change in attitude. This change is very important, although it's not as conspicuous as changes in behavior. The simple acknowledgment "I really do have a problem," or "This eating disorder is ruining my life," is a monumental change in your perception that allows you to consider recovery as an option. It is a wonderful feeling, and only with positive changes in attitude such as this can lasting changes in behavior occur. Seeing

One story of recovery

"I needed to first of all turn my search for answers inward. I kept blaming my lack of control on certain situations (such as potluck dinners, or being around desserts), and on problems outside myself. I also thought that if I only became thin enough I wouldn't have any problems any more, and consequently I wouldn't binge. I discovered that I needed to work from the inside out—I had to let go of all the emotions I'd been stuffing down and learn to love myself for who I was, as I was.

"I also needed support. I told a few friends about my bingeing and I took a workshop for women. The workshop was about self-esteem and general life issues, not eating disorders, but it gave me a safe place to discuss my disorder and deal with bottled-up pain. I cried from beginning to end, almost. I felt very free and almost euphoric. We formed support groups that met once a week—this provided the ongoing support I needed. Believe it or not, I never again binged after that weekend. I turned to my friends and support group instead of to food. I believe that letting myself cry while being supported was the very thing I needed, and the very thing I had been avoiding."

your success and your improving behavior, such as vomiting less or being able to add some food to your daily intake, improves your attitude even further, bringing feelings of "I can do it again. I am proud of my accomplishment. Recovery *is* possible."

Using the Ripple Effect

Because there are so many contributing and complicating factors in eating disorders, it often seems as if there is a mountain of issues to work on, and that it's a task too overwhelming to attempt. The person with the eating disorder—and her family and friends—may feel that all they've been given is a spoon to dig through this mountain of difficulty! But putting time and effort into any one of the issues often has a ripple effect. Lifting depression (perhaps with medication or therapy) can make dealing with eating-disorder goals or life problems in general more manageable. Working to decrease bingeing may have a positive influence on moods and relationships. If you don't tackle all the factors at once, but work on a few at a time, your success in one area may influence other areas.

Another useful image is that of a demolition process. The largest demolition project in the world took place in Calgary, Canada, in 1998. Fifteen hospital buildings spread over several city blocks were brought down at the same moment by implosion, using a few carefully placed explosives. An implosion is a burst of energy directed *inward*. The explosives had only a millionth of the weight of the hospital structures, yet they were enough to bring these massive buildings down. In the same way, well-planned treatment or self-help efforts can make the whole eating-disorder structure collapse from the inside.

How Long Does Recovery Take?

The time varies significantly from person to person, even when two people share a similar history and treatment strategy. It can range from a few months to several years. It's important *not* to set a rigid time-frame; accept that treatment will take as long as it takes. You have the time. The goal is worth it. When you are discouraged about how long progress seems to be taking, look back again and identify the improvements you have already made.

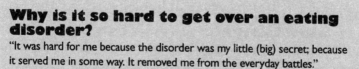

Why is it so hard to get over an eating disorder?

"It was hard for me because the disorder was my little (big) secret; because it served me in some way. It removed me from the everyday battles."

"It meant letting go of my best friend."

"I was so afraid of getting fat. Even if I got to the average weight for my age and height, I would think I was fat."

"It owned me."

The Risks of Recovery

Recovery is not easy; it means letting go of all you have held valuable in the eating disorder. You will have to face the anxiety of changing your eating pattern and giving up any and all eating-disorder behaviors. You may face the further anxiety brought on by weight gain. You will lose your identity as "a person with an eating disorder." You will be expected to interact with people from whom you may have been isolating yourself. You risk becoming your own person and having to make your own way in the world. You will have to make choices, and although they will eventually lead you to fulfillment, along the way there will be disappointments and failures. You must accept all of these as you work toward becoming the primary determiner of your own life journey.

Do I Need Formal Treatment or Can I Make It on My Own?

If your eating disorder has not been a problem for a long time and has not been severe, you may recover spontaneously, without treatment. But while it is not impossible for someone with a long-standing eating disorder to recover alone, this is fairly rare. The longer the eating disorder has had control of your life, the more difficult it will be for you to re-establish control without seeking outside help. Statistics on recovery without treatment are not available, but—as a rule—recovery involves some form of treatment from professionals as well as your own self-help efforts. The goal of such treatment is to allow you to take control of your eating-disorder attitudes and behaviors yourself. Treatment programs do not give you this control; they just help you arrive at your goal sooner. Professionals can only help you, they can't cure you. They help you identify strengths within yourself, so that you can find your own path to recovery.

Why Do People Resist Treatment?

The same factors that led to the eating disorder can create resistance to recovery. Even when you really want to recover, established attitudes and behaviors are strong habits that are difficult to break. Some people make impressive progress, yet can't seem to let go of the eating disorder completely. Habits—whether chewing your nails, smoking cigarettes or behaviors specifically related to eating disorders—need special attention, and there are behavioral techniques that can help you free your life from such ingrained patterns.

The Two-Track Approach

The two-track theory states that you can focus on recovery from the eating disorder and still participate in routine life events. In other words, it says that you can work on your eating disorder and also get on with life—working, going to school and so on—at the same time. However, sometimes it's necessary to take one track at a time, since tackling the eating disorder and being at work or school may be too much to handle at once. Sometimes the fastest way to get back to a normal life is to put the eating-disorder treatment first for a while, and leave the rest of your life on hold. If you take a few months or even a year to focus on recovery, you may save yourself years of suffering. Recovery takes a lot of commitment, and without this commitment—and the focus it demands—working toward a normal life may be extremely difficult.

Time for a Break

Working on an eating disorder is very draining for the person with the disorder, as well as for family members and professional caregivers. Sometimes, when you are at an impasse in treatment, it's wise to take time out from focusing on recovery. Even when progress seems evident, breaks from treatment

What helps?

"I met a man who helped me feel my worth and changed my thinking around to a positive way. I also realized I don't have to act on negative feelings. I think I was ready, and he was the impetus I needed. Now I'm doing it for myself, but he was there for me long enough. I became able to depend on myself as reason enough to remain committed."

"The most important thing that made me turn around my eating disorder was learning to trust and accept myself, and my reactions to life around me."

"If I have turned around for the better, and I guess I have a little bit (I'm not purging breakfast, and I'm bingeing less), it's because I have finally found a doctor who understands my problem, one I can talk to without feeling embarrassed. Also, I know what my eating disorder can do to my body, and I don't want to make it worse."

should be viewed as necessary periods of healing and adjustment, of rejuvenation, and not as wasted time or stalling.

In the case of eating-disorder treatment, much of the healing and recovery happens *between periods of active treatment*, when the body and the mind have a chance to absorb and act upon the advances made during treatment. Too much intense effort all at once or for too long may only work against the process. The changes you are attempting are significant and the pressures on you are great. Sometimes it helps to take a rest.

When Nothing Seems to Be Working

There may be times when nothing seems to move your recovery ahead. There may be no visible progress for months, or things may actually be getting worse. These are times of great frustration for everyone. Some people blame others for the lack of progress. Some go looking for another treatment option. Others feel that it's time to give up altogether.

This is when everyone—the person with the eating disorder, and her supporters, both personal and professional—should regroup and discuss where the recovery process has led to date. It's often helpful to see that progress has in fact been made, at least in the past. Then, discuss the likely reasons why progress has stalled. If possible solutions can be identified, they allow you a new approach. If no reasonable solutions come to light, it may be time to halt active treatment for a while, providing there are no serious health risks that need urgent attention. It may simply be necessary to change the focus of treatment. For example, if efforts to improve nutrition as well as to control bingeing, purging, exercise compulsion and vomiting are not effective, consider directing treatment toward controlling only one behavior (such as vomiting). You may have been trying to change too many things at one time.

A lack of obvious progress doesn't necessarily mean that things aren't changing for the better. Progress may be happening at a subconscious level, and may soon manifest itself—first as a change in attitude, and then as changes in behaviors. Months of seeming lack of progress can end with a sudden awareness of the focus of treatment, and an apparently rapid progression. That's when you realize that you were traveling down the road to recovery all the time.

Will My Eating Disorder Return?

Many people who have an eating disorder want to know, "Will it come back after I finish treatment?" The honest answer to this question is that no one knows for sure, but more treatment is always available. It is possible that certain stressors will bring back the old feelings and patterns. You may feel the eating disorder tugging at you, sending you signals. During these periods, it's natural to fear that the disorder will return. This healthy, normal fear triggers strong defenses to protect you against re-entering the world of eating disorders.

If you ever feel that you are at risk this way, remember that you were able to pull yourself out of the disorder before and you will be able to do so again. All the skills you used to recover are still within and around you, and are readily available if you need them again.

Some people ask, "Can I consider myself truly recovered or am I really a bulimic [or anorexic] for life, just as many recovered alcoholics feel they are alcoholics for life?" Most professionals involved with eating disorders feel that you should accept yourself as truly recovered once the eating disorder has been dealt with. If the old attitudes and behaviors return, remind yourself, "I am someone who has recovered from an eating disorder and I am just having a setback." Remember, you are now in control.

What Have I Learned from My Eating Disorder?

At first glance, this may seem like a ridiculous question. Those who have had an eating disorder typically feel that they have wasted a lot of their life, and that the whole experience has no positive aspects. All they can remember are difficult times that never seemed to end. They lament the lost time, relationships, educational and employment options and happiness.

But surviving an eating disorder often brings unique opportunities for self-discovery and enlightenment. Surprising as it seems, it may actually make you a better person. Relationships within your family may have strengthened. You may have been able to connect with a spouse, parent or sibling in a positive way that was not possible before. You may have learned how to take charge in relationships and take charge of your life, and how to distance yourself from people you cannot change. You will have learned what personal strengths you have, and discovered that what you perhaps thought of as weaknesses are indeed worthwhile characteristics. You may

Thinking back

"When I was immersed in my eating disorder I was clinging to a false sense of control over my body, my life, and the lives of others whom I refused to admit I could not control or protect. The disorder caused me pain, alienation, loneliness and an emotional numbness that made me unable to feel my accomplishments or to achieve happiness."

have learned what you can change in life and what you can't, what is important to you and what isn't. You may have learned to put others' expectations and demands in the proper perspective. You will surely have let go of some of the influences that once held you back or directed you into the eating-disorder pattern.

People who recover from an eating disorder discover these valuable lessons of life much earlier than others. Many people in our society don't travel the path of self-discovery until they are in their thirties, forties, fifties or even older; they don't learn how to cope with difficult life experiences or major personal loss until that time. In contrast, you will be able to call upon your strengths much more quickly, and you are more aware of what you can do to empower yourself. You have the potential to be happy.

What You Can Do to Help Yourself

An essential part of recovery is accepting any treatment option that you may have denied yourself. If therapy, medical monitoring, nutrition services, an eating-disorders program, self-help groups, or medication or drug and alcohol programs are reasonable options, engage in any treatment that seems promising. The help of others can be an invaluable piece of your recovery process. Remember that *you* are making the choice to accept treatment.

Things you can do to avoid reminders of weight issues

- Throw away tight clothing and buy looser garments.
- Hide, cover up or avoid mirrors.
- Hide, give away or throw away your scales.
- Don't buy magazines with advertisements of underweight models.
- Turn off the television during mealtime, to avoid food and diet advertisements.
- Stay away from people who make thinness and dieting an issue.
- Avoid gyms.

Do as much as you can on your own, too. Writing in a journal, keeping eating-activity records or writing meal plans, setting goals, doing visualization exercises, reading self-help books (bibliotherapy), learning from others who have experienced an eating disorder, collecting affirmations or meditating may be of help. So may relaxation exercises, religious faith, or simply having fun! Some self-help projects can be shared with your therapist, your nutritionist or a family member.

Writing in a Journal

A journal or diary is a collection of personal writings, drawings and/or objects. Your writing may be in the form of free thoughts, poetry or letters, or it may simply document what has happened each day. You can write down goals, wish lists and personal aspirations. This provides a way for you to express your thoughts openly without having to share them with others. Thoughts and emotions of a very personal nature are released from your mind onto paper, helping you free yourself of their influence.

Writing can help you identify emotions that you were unaware of. It also challenges you to put into words the complicated combination of feelings you have within you. Just by doing this, you identify and describe the way you are feeling (and the reason for it). This allows you to begin to deal with these feelings. The process may sound difficult, but it often helps immensely. If you question what your writing represents, you may want to share it with your therapist, who may be able to help you understand it.

Writing can be a way of sharing your thoughts and feelings with others when you cannot bring yourself to do so by speaking directly. Sometimes writing and then throwing away your own words is a symbolic letting go, allowing you to cast off an unwanted part of your life—your eating disorder, or any other undesirable life event. Writing can also be of value when you reflect on it at a later date. If the process brings painful feelings, sadness or even depression, share this with your therapist—or just stop writing. Only write if there is likely to be a positive outcome of one sort or another.

You can also sketch or draw in your journal, or tape or paste in objects. You can add magazine clippings, letters from others, food labels or pieces of cloth—all kinds of things. The artwork can be private or you can share it with your therapist.

Eating-Activity Records

Eating-activity records are used to record not only what you eat and drink in a day but also what your eating-disorder behaviors, attitudes and feelings are on a daily basis. You can record the time of day, whom you are eating with and where you are eating. Note your emotions before, during and after eating or bingeing and purging. The eating-activity record helps you identify the relationship between eating and your behaviors, and the emotions that are associated with them and even drive them. By clarifying these associations, and the possible effect of your emotions upon your behavior, you can begin to see the pattern of these behaviors and feelings. This is often the first step in recovery.

Meal Plans

A meal plan is a guide to help you return to a healthier eating pattern. It is a way to lay out reasonable and predictable food choices on a day-to-day or week-to-week basis. It takes away the anxiety of choosing foods at every single meal, thus decreasing stress. It can be compared to a road map directing you toward your eating goals. Your nutritionist or therapist can help you create meal plans, and eventually you may be able to create them for yourself. The meal plan can act as a kind of contract with your caregivers, about your mutually-agreed-upon food choices.

Meal plans not only let you identify food choices and quantities but also allow you to plan the timing of snacks and meals. They must be tailor-made to suit your daily schedule and state of recovery.

Setting Goals

Setting simple, achievable goals is a way of getting started in treatment. Goals help you focus treatment and set aside things that interfere with recovery. They help you prioritize your treatment options. They may or may not be related to your eating disorder.

Eating-disorder goals are such things as adding a couple of portions to your meal plan, decreasing vomiting from three times a day to twice daily, meeting a short-term, realistic weight-gain goal or decreasing the number of diet pills taken weekly.

Other goals are just as important. Decreasing your extracurricular activities, increasing your contacts with friends and family, cutting down on work hours, confronting your partner about an issue that upsets you, or simply having more fun are all common goals.

Goals should be simple and realistic. Go slowly. If you binge twice a day, a dramatic change such as "I will not binge

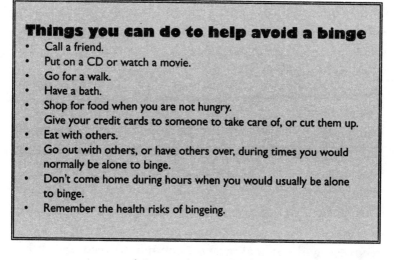

Things you can do to help avoid a binge
- Call a friend.
- Put on a CD or watch a movie.
- Go for a walk.
- Have a bath.
- Shop for food when you are not hungry.
- Give your credit cards to someone to take care of, or cut them up.
- Eat with others.
- Go out with others, or have others over, during times you would normally be alone to binge.
- Don't come home during hours when you would usually be alone to binge.
- Remember the health risks of bingeing.

even once next week" may be too ambitious; set a goal of bingeing only once daily, or just once during one day in the next week.

Goals are targets to test your readiness for making a specific change, not guarantees that you are able to make that change. If you can meet your goal, that is very positive. If you can't, try again, or make your goal a little more reasonable, or wait a while. Don't see not achieving your goal as a failure or an opportunity for self-criticism; see it as a practice run,

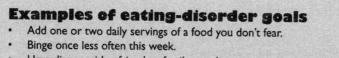

Examples of eating-disorder goals
- Add one or two daily servings of a food you don't fear.
- Binge once less often this week.
- Have dinner with a friend or family member.
- Take half the pills (diuretics, laxatives, diet pills) you would usually take daily.
- See your therapist or nutritionist.
- Go to an eating-disorders support group.
- Exercise less today.
- Avoid someone who makes you feel bad about yourself.
- Take medications that you know have helped you.

and an opportunity to learn. The only people who don't have difficulty achieving goals are those who don't have goals! Working on goals is like learning to play the piano; repeated practice brings rewards.

Visualization

Sometimes, to make something desirable happen, it's important to imagine that it *can* happen, or to imagine what life would be like if it *did* happen. To move forward in recovery, it may be important to imagine what recovery would feel like. This makes the possibility seem more tangible. It may also help you avoid false expectations. It puts you in the mind-set of recovery without making you commit to recovery. What would it be like not to have to focus all that energy on eating and purging? What would your relationship with friends and family be like if you didn't have an eating disorder? What would it be like to go to school or hold a job? How would you look? Visualization is a safe way to experience a life of recovery. Your therapist may be able to help you with visualization exercises, and to discuss your imagined picture of what recovery would be like.

Bibliotherapy

"Bibliotherapy" simply means reading material that helps your recovery. Many self-help books explain the particulars of eating disorders, and suggest treatment tasks or exercises. They may suggest other reading material. Some books and articles give personal accounts of individuals who have experienced an eating disorder, and what recovery was like for them. There are also books for families, written by parents and therapists. See the list provided at the end of this book.

Bibliotherapy allows you to work on your eating disorder on your own time and at your own pace. You can select what is important for you and leave the rest alone. Bibliotherapy may also be appropriate while you work with a therapist; often the material is a good focus for discussion.

Learning from Recovered Individuals

It's easier to believe in recovery, to visualize it, if you know stories of recovery. Eating-disorder associations and support groups can provide you with access to people who have recovered. There are several books with first-hand stories of recovery, and self-help videos often feature recovered anorexics or bulimics recounting their own recovery process.

Affirmations

Affirmations are brief statements that allow you to develop a positive and kind attitude toward yourself as you recover. They are usually one short sentence or phrase that can be expressed anytime, anywhere. You can create the affirmations yourself, copy them from books or take them away from therapy sessions. They help you change by emphasizing your positive traits rather than your negative ones. There are even books that provide an affirmation for each day.

Meditation

Meditation techniques help to relax both the mind and the body. They may or may not have a spiritual component. There are many forms of meditation, and they all allow you some

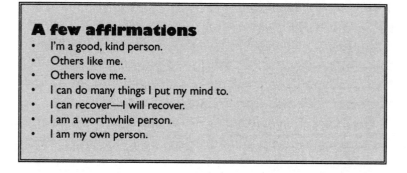

A few affirmations
- I'm a good, kind person.
- Others like me.
- Others love me.
- I can do many things I put my mind to.
- I can recover—I will recover.
- I am a worthwhile person.
- I am my own person.

time away from the stresses of life with an eating disorder. Your therapist may meditate with you, or suggest techniques you can try on your own, or you can learn meditation practices from books. Meditation often gives you back some sense of control over your life, as well as some peace.

Relaxation Exercises

Relaxation exercises are used to decrease stress. There are various techniques and approaches, and you can follow them alone, with your therapist or in groups. Relaxation tapes are readily available to help you learn and then practice the technique. Massage therapy, yoga and tai chi may be useful for relaxation. You can also learn techniques from books, or by signing up for a course.

Religious Faith

Religious faith in one form or another is often helpful in the course of recovery. It may provide an inner resolve and optimism that you have not found elsewhere. Consider whether you have overlooked this as a source of strength.

Have Fun!

Most people with eating disorders have lost the ability to enjoy themselves. Learning to have fun again should be a primary goal of recovery. Ordinary obligations such as working, going to school and studying leave little room for anything else in a day; with an eating disorder and depression, having fun may be a distant memory. Fun can even seem like a frivolous or purposeless endeavor not worthy of your energy, or something you feel you don't deserve. But without fun, all of life's demands, including recovery, are just hard work.

Fun helps to lighten the heart. It rejuvenates us and gives us a reason to get up in the morning, and something to look forward to in the day. Fun provides a purpose for recovery, something to aim for. As eating disorders rob you of the joy of life, fun helps bring it back.

Fun should not involve any tasks that make you feel that you are in competition with others, or that you must meet their expectations. It should be uplifting, not a burden. Fun should not be work! It should also be easily obtainable and immediate, not something you might do next year. Planning enjoyment for the future may be a good thing, but make sure you are also going to have fun now.

A Story of Hope and Recovery

"I learned at a young age that it was wrong to cry, and that getting angry meant major blowups. Basically I avoided conflict at all cost, liking what others liked and agreeing with whatever anyone said. Expecting perfection from myself, I was constantly let down. I had no self-esteem and no idea who I was.

"To gain some control of my life, I began not eating, off and on, in my teens. After high school my eating disorder progressed as a result of a bad relationship with a man. My grandfather was sick, my mom and stepdad were returning to town, and my dad and twin sister weren't getting along. I wanted to die.

"I drank hot mustard and water to make myself sick, and I abused laxatives, taking several at a time. I lost a lot of weight in two months. I had four thousand dollars in the bank and I was going to move out of my parents' home so I could be by myself and not eat, but that didn't happen. Then I gained some weight. Over the next few years I was in and out of hospital, each time gaining weight and, upon release, losing weight again. One night I even took an overdose. Well, I didn't die.

"My weight was okay for a year before my mother's suicide. One and a half years later I was back in hospital for the last time. There I let myself grieve and I made a decision: I would either live without the disorder, which had become my identity, or I would die. I chose to live.

"I have started to take control of my life by saying no and not always agreeing with everyone. Learning to cry and get angry has helped me immensely. I'm married now, I have two children, and I'm determined not to let the eating disorder return. I am still discovering who I am.

"My belief is that anyone can overcome an eating disorder. You just have to take control of your life and deal with the cause of the disorder, not only the symptoms. A support system is also very important. I'm 29 years old but my life has just begun, and I plan on living it to the fullest."

A Final Word

With all the challenges that an eating disorder brings to you as well as your family and friends, it's important to know that recovery is possible. Just by reading this book you are working on recovery. Whatever doubts you may have, make the most of the resources listed at the end of this book. Use all the resources available to you, but always remember—*you* are your own greatest resource. You are in control.

Table of Drug Names

Generic name	Some common brand names	Used for
Tricyclics		
amitriptyline	Elavil	depression
desipramine	Norpramin	
imipramine	Tofranil	
nortriptyline	Aventyl, Pamelor*	
SSRIs		
fluoxetine	Prozac	depression and anxiety
fluvoxamine	Luvox	
paroxetine	Paxil	
sertraline	Zoloft	
citalopram	Celexa	
SNRI◆		anxiety
venlafaxine	Effexor	depression and anxiety
Antipsychotic		
olanzapine	Zyprexa	decreased rumination about body image and weight fears
Benzodiazepines		
clonazepam	Klonopin*, Rivotril†	anxiety
diazepam	Valium	
flurazepam	Dalmane	
lorazepam	Ativan	
oxazepam	Serax	
Motility modifiers		
domperidone	Motilium†	gastric distress
metoclopramide	Reglan	

◆ SNRI=Serotonin Norepinephrine Reuptake Inhibitor
* U.S.A. only
† Canada only

Glossary

Amenorrhea: absence of normal menstrual period.

Binge: a period of rapid, uncontrolled overeating.

Bipolar disorder: a disorder of mood or emotion in which depression alternates with mania (high energy and euphoria) or irritability; also called manic-depressive disorder.

Cachexia: profound weight loss.

Calorie: *see* **Kilocalorie.**

Cheilosis: painful cracks in the corners of the mouth that may be caused by vomiting.

Compulsion: recurring urges to perform a certain behavior.

Diuretic: a chemical that causes a person to produce more urine than usual.

Edema: swelling caused by accumulation of excess fluid in a part of the body.

Electrolytes: essential chemicals (such as sodium and potassium) found in body fluids; often thrown out of balance in eating disorders.

Emaciation: marked weight loss.

Emetic: a substance swallowed to induce vomiting.

Esophagus: the tube that connects the mouth to the stomach.

Hyperphagia: overeating.

Kilocalorie: a measure of the energy in food. "Kilocalorie" is the scientific term; it is often shortened to "calorie."

Kwashiorkor: a medical condition characterized by muscle wasting, accumulation of excess fluid in the legs and a swollen abdomen, caused by starvation, particularly lack of protein.

Lanugo: fine, down-like hairs that appear on the face and body in anorexia nervosa.

Mallory-Weiss tears: tears in the esophagus, produced by forceful or repeated vomiting.

Metabolic rate: a measure of how active and efficient the body is in producing energy.

Metabolism: all the chemical and physical processes involved in the body's production of energy.

Nasogastric: involving the nose and stomach. In nasogastric feeding, a tube carries liquid nutrients through the nose and esophagus to the stomach.

Obese: very overweight.

Obsession: a recurring intrusive thought, feeling or idea.

Oropharynx: the back of the throat, which can be stimulated to induce vomiting.

Osteoporosis: a disease of thinning or loss of density in the bones.

Purge: in eating disorders, to deliberately eliminate food from the stomach and/or bowel by vomiting, laxatives, etc.

Refeeding: increasing someone's food intake, and helping the person establish a more normal eating pattern.

Reflux: the passage of acid and other stomach contents upward into the esophagus and sometimes into the mouth.

Restricting: in eating disorders, severe limiting of food choices and amounts.

Satiation: a normal feeling of stomach fullness.

Satiety: the feeling of not being hungry, which results from a number of factors.

Seasonal affective disorder: cyclic depression that commonly occurs during winter months, when sunlight is diminished.

Signs: physical changes (such as weight loss) that can be observed by another person.

Symptoms: physical changes (such as headache) that are not apparent to another person.

Syndrome: a group of symptoms and signs that characterize a disease or disorder.

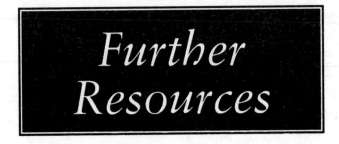

Further Resources

Organizations

United States

Academy for Eating Disorders (AED)
6728 Old McLean Village Drive
McLean, VA 22101
(703) 556-9222
Fax: (703) 556-8729
aed@degnon.org
www.acadeatdis.org

American Anorexia Bulimia Association, Inc. (AABA)
165 West 46th Street
Suite 1108
New York, NY 10036
(212) 575-6200
info@aabainc.org
www.aabainc.org

National Eating Disorders Association
603 Stewart St., Suite 803
Seattle, WA 98101
(206) 382-3587
Fax: (206) 829-8501
Toll-free: 1-800-931-2237 (U.S. only)
www.nationaleating disorders.org

Harvard Eating Disorders Center
℅ Massachusetts General Hospital WACC-7275
15 Parkman St.
Boston, MA 02114
(617) 236-7766
www.hedc.org

National Association of
Anorexia Nervosa and
Associated Disorders
(ANAD)
P.O. Box 7
Highland Park, IL 60035
(847) 831-3438
Fax: (847) 433-4632
www.anad.org

We Insist on Natural Shape
(WINS)
P.O. Box 19938
Sacramento, CA 95819
Toll-free:1-800-600-9467
(U.S. only)
www.winsnews.org

Canada

Bridgepoint Centre for
Eating Disorders
P.O. Box 190
Milden, SA S0L 2L0
(306) 935-2240
bridgepoint@sk.sympatico.ca
www.saskworld.com/
holistic/bridgepoint
(Specializes in adolescents
and adults)

Vancouver Island Association
for Ending Disordered
Eating (VIAEDE)
(formerly the British
Columbia Eating
Disorders Association)
525 Michigan Street
Victoria, BC V8V 1S2
(250) 383-2755
Fax: (250) 383-5518
viaede@look.ca
www.preventingdisordered
eating.org

Bulimia Anorexia Nervosa
Association (BANA)
300 Cabana Road E.
Windsor, ON N9G 1A3
(519) 969-2112
Fax: (519) 969-0227
www.bana.ca

Eating Disorders Resource
Centre of British
Columbia
4500 Oak Street
(Women's Health Centre
Building)
Room E200, Mailbox 134
Vancouver, BC V6H 3N1
(604) 875-2084
Fax: (604) 875-3688
Toll-free: 1-800-665-1822
(B.C. only)
edrcbc@direct.ca

Eating Disorders Program
Maritime Outpatient
  Psychiatry
IWK Health Centre
5850 University Avenue
Halifax, NS B3J 3G9
(902) 470-8375
Fax: (902) 470-8937

Hospital for Sick Children
Eating Disorders Program
555 University Avenue
Toronto, ON M5G 1X8
(416) 813-7195
Fax: (416) 813-7867
www.sickkids.on.ca
(For people under 19)

National Eating Disorder
  Information Centre
  (NEDIC)
200 Elizabeth Street
Toronto, ON M5G 2C4
(416) 340-4156
Fax: (416) 340-4736
Toll-free: 1-866-NEDIC-20
www.nedic.ca
*(The NEDIC website
supplies a comprehensive
list of other organizations.)*

Sheena's Place
87 Spadina Road
Toronto, ON M5R 2T1
(416) 927-8900
www.sheenasplace.org

Books

Fairburn, Christopher. *Overcoming Binge Eating.* New York, NY: Guilford Press, 1995.

Hall, Lindsey. *Full Lives.* Carlsbad, CA: Gürze Books, 1993.

———, and Leigh Cohn. *Bulimia: A Guide to Recovery.* Carlsbad, CA: Gürze Books, 1992.

Johnston, Anita A. *Eating in the Light of the Moon.* Secaucus, NJ: Birch Lane Press, 1996.

Miller, Scott D., Barry L. Duncan and Mark A. Hubble. *Escape from Babel.* New York, NY: W. W. Norton & Company, 1996.

Normandi, Carol Emery, and Laurelee Roark. *It's Not about Food.* New York, NY: Grosset/Putnam, 1998.

Schwartz, Mark F., and Leigh Cohn. *Sexual Abuse and Eating Disorders.* New York, NY: Brunner/Mazel, 1996.

Siegel, Michelle, Judith Brisman and Margo Weinshel. *Surviving an Eating Disorder: Strategies for Family and Friends.* New York, NY: Harper Perennial, 1997.

Index